JESUS WAS HERE

(More Lasagna, Please)
Feeding the Soul of a Grieving Mother

Michelle Bauer
Skrive Publications
Miramar Beach, FL
U.S.A.

Copyright © 2020 by Michelle Bauer

All rights reserved

No part of this book may be transmitted or reproduced in any form by any means without permission from the publisher.

A portion of the proceeds from the sale of each book will be donated to the Beyond Type 1 program called *Jesse Was Here*. If you would like to donate: www.jesse-was-here.org

Printed in the U.S.A.

Cover design by Liz Nitardy

ISBN 978-1-952037-19-1 (Paperback)
ISBN 978-1-952037-18-4 (eBook)

SKRIVE PUBLICATIONS
Miramar Beach, FL
608-332-6986
www.skrivepublications.com

Reviews

This book was given to me as a gift. *Jesse Was Here* is a poignant, heartfelt, insightful, necessary read. I would recommend it to anyone who is grieving the loss of a loved one, especially because of illness. Michelle is an incredible T1D advocate and champion. She has put so much care and heart into this story – her story. It takes courage to share one that is so personal. She is a giver! This book isn't just about grief but finding a way to heal.

Julia

I met Michelle and her husband, Jeff, at a JDRF ride many years ago. I immediately became extended family, yet I feel closer to them having read this remarkable tribute to and continued celebration of Jesse's life. He was such a cool, extroverted and remarkable young man. Jesse and my late brother, Bobby, (died at age 36, from T1D complications as well on 12-25-02), were very much alike and both gone far too soon. As I continue to process my own losses, I will always be grateful to Michelle for sharing her compelling and uplifting story, especially how she was able to find joy in the face of tragedy. Thank you, Michelle!

Eric

In the normal course of events, our children are the legacies we leave to the world. In an often cruel world, parents sometimes outlive their children. With her book, *Jesse Was Here*, Michelle Bauer has become the keeper of her son's legacy here on earth. This journal of a mom's journey moving forward after grief is inspiring and heart wrenching. Her willingness to share her vulnerabilities and struggles over the decade since Jesse died is part of that legacy. There is something to be learned in *Jesse Was Here* for anyone who has lost someone they love or is supporting someone who has lost a loved one. Michelle's writing is engaging and intimate. Jesse *was* here, and anyone reading this book will be touched by his legacy.

Janet

People say, "It takes a village to raise a child." This read proves it takes a village to grieve one as well. This thought-provoking read not only helps put into perspective the grief of a parent but that of the village. As a card carrying lasagna supplier, I appreciated this book so much and feel a little more prepared as a village member!

Erin

MICHELLE BAUER

Grief is one of those things you don't really want to talk about or read about. However, death is part of life and being better prepared to deal with it is important. Michelle is one of those people who is always helping others, so when she lived through the unimaginable experience of the death of her son, she knew she was in a unique position to help other people who are struggling. Through this book she shows there is no right or wrong way to grieve. She points out that everyone's grief is different. Her list of *Things Not to Say* and her *Guide for Family and Friends* are particularly powerful. Very useful information for anyone that wants to help someone through difficult times.

Robin

Dedication

To Samantha and Joey, my reasons for getting out of bed and tying my shoes each of those dark days

Contents

PUBLISHER'S NOTE 11

FOREWORDS 15

AUTHOR'S NOTE 23

1 - Purpose (Six months after Jesse's death) 25
2 - Wednesday is Just Wednesday (One year after Jesse's death) 31
3 - Whatever Works (One month after Jesse's death) 39
4 - Shopping at Target (Two months after Jesse's death) 53
5 - Dealing with the Dingleberries (Three months after Jesse's death) 57
6 - Everyone Grieves Differently (Four months after Jesse's death) 61
7 - Turning a Corner (Four months after Jesse's death) 71
8 - Since Everything Happened (Five months after Jesse's death) 79

9 - An Ambulance is Just an Ambulance (Six months after Jesse's death)..........................95

10 - The Holidays – Anything But Merry (10 Months, 14 days after Jesse's death)..........................105

11 - Intimacy, Relationships, Beginnings, Endings (Five Years After Jesse's death)....................115

12 - The Worst Day of My Life (Six months after Jesse's death) 123

13 - Compartmentalized Living (Five years after Jesse's death) 151

14 - I Don't Care That Your Cat Died (Written over a period of time after Jesse's death)................... 157

15 - How Many Kids do you Have? (Written over several months following Jesse's death) 167

16 - A Guide for Family and Friends (Written over time after Jesse's death).....................................175

HOW JESSE WAS HERE CAME TO BE 181
EPILOGUE.. 185
RESOURCES 189
JDRF RIDE TO CURE DIABETES 193
MEMORIES... 197
LIFE SENTENCE BY JOE BRADY 205
ABOUT THE AUTHOR 207

Publisher's Note

I MET MICHELLE BAUER IN MADISON, WISCONSIN, in 2005, when she was director of the local chapter of the Juvenile Diabetes Research Foundation (JDRF). Our youngest son had been diagnosed with type 1 diabetes as an 8-year-old in 1996. Her son Jesse had been diagnosed with the same disease in March of 2000, so we had something in common. We did a lot of fundraising for JDRF at the time, and I had stopped by her office to drop off some cash and checks. We chatted for a bit and discovered that we were both involved in the local triathlon community as well. I had just completed my first Ironman in 2004 and she was training for her first attempt at Ironman in 2006.

We would see each other occasionally at her office and at triathlons around the area. She and Jesse had become tireless advocates for people in the diabetes community. My wife and I were saddened to hear that Jesse died unexpectedly in February of 2010 from complications related to his diabetes. It was a devastating event for Michelle and her family and, as you might suspect, it resonated deeply with our family as well.

We stayed in touch for a period of time after that, including the years she worked for *Brava* magazine. *Brava* had planned to do a feature on my wife and her business success, and Michelle was instrumental in directing that project. In 2014, my wife and I relocated from Wisconsin to Florida and I lost touch with Michelle. We did, however, remain friends on social media.

In February, 2020, I saw that Michelle had posted a question on her Facebook page. She wanted suggestions for a good new book to read. Having recently started my own publishing company, Skrive Publications, I commented on her timeline and suggested she read one of my books!

She called me a few minutes later and said, "Dan, I think you might be the answer to my prayers!"

Michelle told me she had started writing a book shortly after Jesse died and had added chapters to the story over the course of the next five years. It was one of the ways she grieved the loss of her son. She had been encouraged by others to get the story published but like many unknown and unpublished writers, she found it difficult to get anybody to look at her manuscript. She submitted it to several different publishing companies. Nobody would even look at it, let alone publish it.

I told her to send the manuscript to me. I'd review it and give her some honest feedback. She sent me everything that she had finished at the time. Honestly, it was raw and a bit unorganized and needed a lot of work. But, like I've always said, "Every story matters." This story matters to her; it matters to me; and I believe it will matter to a lot of people who have children with type 1 diabetes or have diabetes themselves. It will especially matter to other parents who have lost children to this disease. I told Michelle that I would be honored to work with her to get her story published.

I was talking to another independent publisher recently. He was excited about a project that he had just finished. He said, "Dan, there's something magical about helping a person bring his or her story to life. It doesn't matter if the published book sells a million copies or just makes the author happy. Every story matters."

My hope is that *Jesse Was Here* will be an inspiring read and a helpful tool for other people who have experienced what Michelle went through. It is raw and real and offers guidance and hope to anybody who has lost a loved one.

Foreword

FEW PEOPLE PERSONIFY NIETZSCHE'S SIMPLE yet profound observation "That which does not kill us makes us stronger" quite like Michelle Bauer.

I first met Michelle in 2013 at the American Diabetes Association's annual conference. I was there because my older daughter had been diagnosed with type 1 diabetes (T1D) in 2007. Five months later, I became a trustee of the Helmsley Charitable Trust (HCT), a multibillion-dollar charitable trust. I came from the business world and didn't understand non-profits or medical research, but I had a strong sense of urgency and even stronger desire to get something done for the T1D community. I knew that Michelle had endured every parent's worst nightmare, losing her son Jesse to T1D. I wanted to talk with her about the circumstances of his death and hear her ideas, but I was nervous about meeting her. I'm not a shy guy, but what could I possibly say to someone who'd experienced such a profound loss?

In 2013, my team and I were still flying below the radar; Helmsley was not that well known in the T1D field, and I liked it that way. There's a joke in philanthropy that you are never wittier, smarter or better-looking than when someone finds out you're a grant-maker, so I used to walk around conferences with my badge turned backward to keep my anonymity. Within two minutes of meeting Michelle, she called me out on this. She not only broke the ice, but I knew right then that we would get along just fine.

As I got to know her, I learned that Michelle is one of the most inspiring, resilient people I had ever met. She turned her catastrophe into her calling – learning from it, growing from it, and most importantly, using her incredibly clear and powerful voice to help others.

A decade after my older daughter was diagnosed with T1D, my younger daughter was diagnosed with the same disease. My wife, my son and I constantly think about the girls' well-being. All parents whose kids have T1D are ridden with constant fear that their children will go to sleep and not wake up, or some other T1D-related tragedy will find us. The hard truth is that T1D is still a killer, but we don't talk about it. It's simply too real and raw. Yet if we don't talk about it, it will keep happening and families will continue to suffer in silence and fear.

Not if Michelle can help it. She has courageously attacked this disease head on. Nobody can understand the trauma, pain and devastation of losing a child unless you have been through it. Michelle is amazingly open about it and serves as a resource for others. This is nothing short of heroic.

I know you will join me with gratitude to Michelle for sharing her story and lending her strength to all of us. I know that you will find her as awe-inspiring as I do.

David Panzirer, Trustee of the Leona M. and Harry B. Helmsley Charitable Trust

Foreword

WHAT TO SAY? WHAT TO SAY? I HAVE known Michelle since my very first JDRF Ride to Cure in 2005 when I rode for the Team Type 1 Foundation. I got the chance to meet Jesse at a JDRF Gala in May of 2008. The boy I met that night was glowing with confidence and happiness in the knowledge that his mother and many, many more people loved him very much.

Michelle took his diagnosis as fuel to drive her to help others and to raise money for diabetes research. It broke my heart to learn of Jesse's passing, and I can only imagine the pain that Michelle and her entire family went through.

However, Michelle powered through and made it one of her life's missions to use her loss as a means to help others, a means to alleviate pain, a means to connect the diabetes community on an even deeper level. Time and time again, Michelle has taken a tremendous challenge and turned it into a chance to help others. She is an inspiration to us all, and I am proud to see her story finally being told here.

If you are in need of inspiration, then dive right into Michelle's story. You'll be stronger for it.

And, Jesse, please know that my 23rd mile is always my best mile, and that is thanks to you, buddy!

Phil Southerland, Founder and CEO, Team Novo Nordisk

Foreword

MARCH 25TH, 2010, WAS EVERY PARENT'S worst nightmare for me and my family. That was the day our 14-year-old son, Trent, died unexpectedly from complications related to type 1 diabetes. I was in a daze, staring, unable to look at or listen to anyone. It was like the world was still moving and I was standing still.

I got a call from a guy named Tom, also known as the Diabetes Dad at Children With Diabetes (CWD), an event that Trent attended each year in Florida. At CWD, we were surrounded by other families living with type 1 diabetes. He was shocked to hear about Trent's death. More importantly, he wanted to tell me that he knew another mom who had just lost her son Jesse a few weeks prior. He thought that maybe we could help each other and asked my permission to give her my number. I remember not being able to even think about talking to her but after some time we started texting and emailing each other. Michelle and I share a life event that bonds us together forever.

Our sons never knew each other, but it feels like they are together looking at us now, enjoying our friendship and giving each other high fives every time we get together or help each other through difficult days. Michelle has been my friend, counselor and voice of reason; she makes me laugh, and she makes me cry! I'm confident I do the same for her as we truly understand each other and move forward together. I am beyond proud of her and am always amazed by her dedication to helping others.

Jen Nicholson, Mother of Trent

Author's Note

MY CURRENT VIEW IS FROM 10 YEARS OUT. It's been that long since my son died. Not a single day has passed that I don't think about Jesse. The hole in my heart will never completely heal. I still miss him today more than anything in the world.

I started writing shortly after Jesse died. It was cathartic for me and helped me relieve some of the anger and anxiety that I experienced. I can't think of anything more unnatural than a parent losing a child. It's not supposed to happen that way. It's backwards and upside down and creates indescribable feelings of guilt and sadness and hopelessness.

Life is for the living, however, and as time passed, I slowly changed. There were times when I thought I'd never be able to move forward from my grief. There were times when I thought I'd never be able to function in a happy, loving relationship again. Thankfully, I was wrong on both counts.

My daughter Samantha and my youngest son Joey stood by me courageously as we walked forward without Jesse. They also brought Jesse's oldest sister, Sara, back into my life in a much bigger and more meaningful way. My husband,

Jeff, loved me unconditionally and brought more joy into my life than I could ever have imagined, not to mention two more amazing kids that I couldn't be more proud to have as part of this crazy blend.

Jesse was Here. That phrase will always hold sad memories for me; however, it has become a well-known mantra in the diabetes community. Even as a young kid, Jesse was a wonderful spokesperson for many people living with type 1 diabetes. I know he'd be pleased that his memory continues to inspire people all over the world.

I'd like to thank Dan Madson and Skrive Publications for taking a chance on me and my story. He was the perfect resource who came into my life at the perfect time. I will always be grateful for the work he and his team did on my behalf.

Finally, I would like to offer a special word of thanks to Sarah Lucas. Sarah was one of the founders of Beyond Type1 and welcomed the program *Jesse Was Here*. She didn't care that it was a scary topic because she realized it was something that people in the diabetes community needed to talk about. She is an amazing, resilient human being who has stood behind me the whole way, even after suffering her own personal obstacles and grief. I will forever be grateful for her help and encouragement.

1
Purpose
(Six months after Jesse's death)

> *"The mystery of human existence lies in not just staying alive, but in finding something to live for."*
> -Fyodor Dostoyevsky

WHEN MY 13-YEAR-OLD SON, JESSE, died unexpectedly on February 3, 2010, from complications related to type 1 diabetes, I felt lost—as lost as any parent on earth whose child has died unexpectedly. Within the first few weeks I tried to find ways to heal even though I quickly came to the realization that I could never heal completely. After Jesse died, I had to find ways to cope, to get out of bed, to live. I spent hours on the Internet searching for books that dealt with grief and bought many of them. I quickly discovered there were many books written by parents who had lost children. There were dozens of books written about Christianity, the soul and life after death. However, I couldn't find anything that I considered to be a realistic look at the feelings I was experiencing. My main thought was simple, "This sucks. This really sucks. This is going to continue to suck, and there's nobody to help me."

I knew I was going to have to help myself. I knew people were going to bring me lasagna even though I didn't want to eat. I knew I would let them do it because it would make them feel better. They were just like me—they didn't know what to do either. I knew that I would find it difficult to ask for help, but I grudgingly realized I should accept help when it was offered.

At first, my goal was to write the details of my first six months of life after Jesse's death. I wanted to share my ups and downs, my bad days and my good days. And there were good days, something I still have a hard time believing. Then it occurred to me to continue writing through that first year. I figured that you and I could grieve together.

As you read this book, especially if you have lost a child, I want you to know it's okay to be ticked off at someone who compares your loss to the death of their cat. I know the person who said that meant well. I want you to know it's okay to grieve by telling the world your every thought while your spouse grieves by not talking about it at all. There are no right or wrong ways to grieve. There was growth that came from that horrible day. I'm already feeling it. I'm trudging forward even when I feel like screaming at the next person who says to me, "I don't know how you do it, Michelle, you're so strong." What the hell was I supposed to do? Crawl into bed and give up on my life?

I could not have written this book if it wasn't for my family and friends. I have an amazing support system surrounding me, helping me, loving me. It's like a fortress. I'm grateful for all of them.

> *I knew people were going to bring me lasagna even though I didn't want to eat.*

To you, friends or family members worried about the right things to say—relax—we will still love you, even if you say something insensitive.

To the reader of this book, especially if you have lost a child, I hope you can experience the same love and support that I've had throughout my journey. Your family and friends love you and want to help. Open up. Let them in.

You are in uncharted territory. Let's get through the first year together.

JESSE WAS HERE

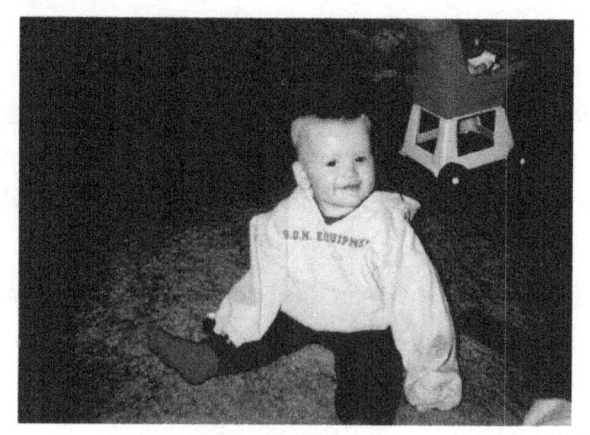

Jesse, age 9 months

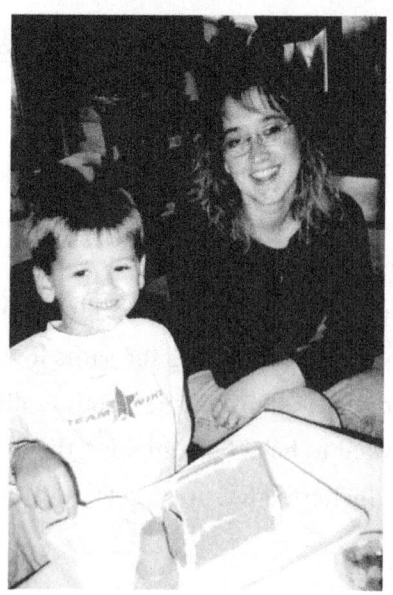

Jesse, age 4, first day of preschool

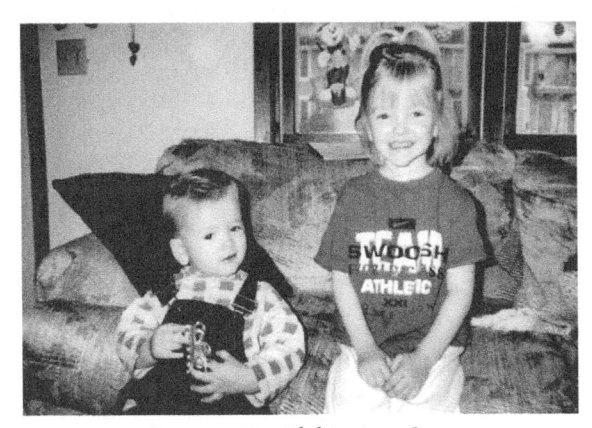

Jesse, age 2, with big sister Sam

2
Wednesday is Just Wednesday

(One year after Jesse's death)

*When one door of happiness closes,
another opens, but often we look so long
at the closed door that we do not see
the one that has been opened for us."
-Helen Keller*

I STARTED WRITING THIS BOOK SHORTLY AFTER Jesse died, and it occurred to me that while I really wanted to focus on the first six months of grief, I wanted to write a follow-up on the exact date of our first anniversary without Jesse. During the first year after Jesse's death I just wanted someone—anyone—to tell me that I would feel something other than pain. I am here to tell you that there is hope and relief.

As I wrote this, there were reminders everywhere of that

fateful day. I had wondered how horrifying that day would be. How I would spend it? Where would I go? Who would I spend it with? I knew I would not be spending the day reliving that horrible nightmare. That slideshow still lurked in the back of my mind. It tried to ooze out on certain days, but on that day I would not torture myself or those around me. Strangely enough, I found that day nowhere near as bad as the hellish month between Thanksgiving and Christmas. That surprised me.

Instead, I spent the day reflecting. One year into my journey without Jesse I discovered little touches of beauty. I recalled trying to explain to others that grief for me was like going through my whole life without seeing the color blue and then suddenly seeing blue everywhere. Or buying a new car and then noticing all the other people who were driving that exact same car. Grief was everywhere, but until you have to fathom the unfathomable, you can't possibly understand other people's grief. Not really. You can try, but I'm here to tell you there's no way to fully understand how others are feeling who have lost a child. God help you, I hope you never have to understand.

Sometime after Jesse's death, I was interviewing a wonderful woman from a national radio show who remembered seeing my story on the news. While telling her about my reference to the color blue she said, "You know, Michelle, blue is a reference to God." So is it okay to see a little bit of God in what has transpired over the last year? For me the answer is yes. For others, it can be whatever they need.

I want to remind you, dear reader, that as you get through your first days, weeks and months and wonder, "Will I ever breathe again?" I'm here to tell you that you will breathe, but your breaths will smart with pain and you will see reminders of your loss everywhere. That is a harsh reality. During those first weeks without Jesse, I could barely get through Wednesdays because Wednesdays were a stark reminder that my son had died a week ago, two weeks ago, three weeks ago. Now? Wednesday is just Wednesday. The relief comes in small steps, one day, one week, one month at a time.

I have a friend named Laura. You'll learn more about her in this book. Her words and guidance got me through those first days, those first months and that first year. She just popped up on my social media one day with this message, "I love you, Michelle, who sees blue now and is beautiful and loving and full of light!"

Her message caused me to pause and reflect that, just like Jesse did in life, in death he brought beautiful people into my life who helped me grow and learn during that first year of my journey. If Jesse were still here, there would be no Laura in my life. She has been a great gift to me.

I often think about the other families I've met who have

lost children to diabetes. These parents are fighters; they are filled with so much love that I can't imagine my life without them. After Jesse died, the diabetes community that I had been part of continued to embrace me. They didn't discard me when I thought I might no longer fit. Instead, I became a resource for many of them. They came to me for advice, no matter how strange I thought it was that they wanted advice from a woman whose son had died. What a gift they have been in this life.

The odd moments continued, but they became easier to handle. One year to the day after Jesse's death, I had a new intern start at the magazine I was working for. Jesse's death remained an awkward thing. I mean, was I supposed to fully disclose his death right away to everybody? Should I not mention it? Was there proper etiquette to explain the death of a child? In any case, my intern popped in to discuss an event we were planning.

We started talking about kids and what kind of music they listened to. I told her how my daughter preferred new music and that my teenage son had liked heavy metal and that my youngest son was still forming an opinion. That conversation turned into a discussion of video games. I sat there uncomfortably, feeling as if I was lying to her by not telling her that my son had died. After all, she was standing across from me listening to me explain my children's tastes in music and video games. Finally I said, "I have this event in the summer in honor of my son. It's called Jessepalooza. Last year for one of the door prizes, we gave away a private tour of Raven Software where they make *Call of Duty*."

Thinking that I was referring to the fact that Jesse had won the door prize, she said, "I bet he just died when he got that!" I knew that moment was going to be more painful for her than for me. I hesitated for a split second and then blurted out, "I'm so sorry, and please do not feel horrified. You couldn't have known this, but my son Jesse died a year ago today." I winced when I saw the look on her face. I'm afraid uncomfortable moments like that will continue to happen until someone writes more clearly about death etiquette.

I thought of my family. Jesse's death brought us together and then tore us apart. We realized throughout that first year that we needed each other and no matter what, we had to stick together. I'm grateful for each of them.

My kids. What can I say here without choking up? My 17-year-old daughter showed so much grace, strength and love that I was in awe of her. Don't get me wrong, I don't want to portray my teenage daughter as perfect. I think that might be against the law. Still, her view of the world overwhelmed me at times. She was not jaded or sad; she was full of life and held onto great memories of Jesse. My 10-year-old son, who went through so much that first year, was my silent one who held all his pain inside. I knew at some point, he would need to seek out someone to talk to. I hoped he would continue to journey in the right direction. I hoped he would continue to remember his brother through stories, videos and good times.

If you are reading this early in your journey of grief, I hope this brings you some comfort as you look at your children and worry about their immediate pain and their futures. You will help get them through. Keep trudging.

> *I often think about the other families I've met who have lost children to diabetes. These parents are fighters; they are filled with so much love that I can't imagine my life without them.*

I wish I could tell you that everything will be OK. I do. But I've learned that grief is a son-of-a-bitch. It can jump up and bite you right in the ass when you least expect it. Sometimes you will have to keep it in line by yourself despite all the best intentions of friends and family. They are not walking in your shoes. My healing continued each and every day, and I wish you the same progress and strength. Who knows? Maybe we can meet again in five years for some more lasagna! I'll bring the garlic bread; you bring the wine.

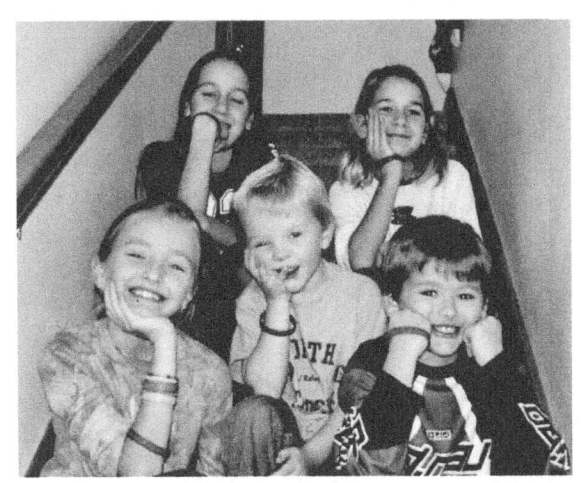

Jesse with neighborhood kids wearing bracelets
that say "Cure Diabetes" that mom made

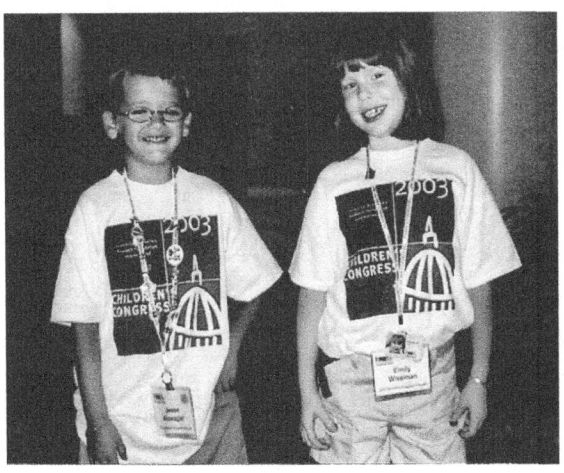

Jesse, age 6, at JDRF Children's Congress
with new friend, Emily

3
Whatever Works

(One month after Jesse's death)

> *"Take a deep breath. Inhale peace. Exhale happiness."*
> *-A.D. Posey*

SO WHO AM I? I WAS RAISED CATHOLIC IN a small town in Wisconsin. I was baptized, I had my first communion, I went to CCD classes – what all the kids did where I lived and grew up. My family wasn't overly religious, but I had a healthy dose of "God doesn't forgive" in my head. When I was in fourth grade, my parents decided to divorce. I remember feeling that our big Catholic church would no longer embrace the collection envelopes from our broken home. It forever changed my opinions about religion.

Don't get me wrong, I don't want to shove my ideas about religion down anybody's throat. It's not why I'm writing this. I only share my perspective on this topic to explain how my background sometimes helped me grieve. At other times it didn't.

Early into adulthood I found the Bible to be a fascinating book. I wanted to read it and form my own perspective without anyone telling me how to interpret its writings. When I read the Bible, I tried to imagine what was going on at the time it was written. Too often, I came away feeling it was a book written by politicians. When I became pregnant for the first time with my daughter, all of those thoughts and feelings entered my head. Should I have her baptized? Would she go to hell if she wasn't? God, the angry judge, was back in my head.

I had switched to an Episcopalian Church (I called it Catholic Light) while pregnant with my first child and gave it a shot as I brought my children into the world as pure little souls – whatever that meant. Father Bill shared with me his thoughts on baptism. As I was going through the teachings of baptism in preparation for my daughter's birth he said, "You know, you don't have to go through with this baptism. You do know children are pure and aren't going to hell, don't you?" Of course I did NOT know that, or I wouldn't have been there. He proceeded to tell me that he believed a baptism should be done when a person was old enough to understand its meaning. That thought stuck with me to this day and has followed me after the loss of my son.

For the next decade or so, I was ambivalent toward religion. Gradually, I started changing my thinking. I decided to look at my religious life as more of a life of spirituality. I had always believed in God, in a higher power. I couldn't believe that this was it for us as humans, or for our souls. I've always believed the body was no more than a garage for the soul, and I never felt particularly close to loved ones who were buried. I always felt you could just feel them, that there was no need to go visit their graves. I didn't really do much about those thoughts as I happily skated through life watching my kids grow up. I didn't realize that all of those things were easy to say until it was my son lying in a hospital bed. It was my son they were asking me about. Did I want a chaplain to come up and perform last rites? Did I want to donate my son's organs? Did I want my son to have an autopsy?

In 2008, I started working for a local women's magazine. While I was working for this magazine, I got to know some interesting people. I came to understand that the world ticks in many different ways. Cynical by nature, I usually spent most of my time looking down my nose at people who talked about "flow massage" or "energy work" or "intuition." After a while, however, I opened myself up to listening to some of those wonderful people and the experiences they had created and shared.

In the fall of 2009, our magazine did an article on a woman who owned a local salon. I heard she had a really great way about her. I heard she was intuitive. Our publisher was wild about this woman and would beam when she talked about her. I could only roll my eyes at the notion. Whenever our magazine went to press and the newly printed copies were delivered to our offices all shiny and colorful, our staff liked to sit down and read them cover to cover. We criticized ourselves, laughed and talked about what was great about the issue and then we'd usually grab a beer afterward. For some reason, while reading this particular issue, I was drawn to the woman who owned the salon. Her photo just spoke to me, "I'm a good person; I don't judge; live your life." I felt compelled to read the feature about her. Sadly, I didn't meet her until quite a while after we featured her. Little did I know that she would become pivotal in the way I handled Jesse's death, the way I handled the funeral and the way I saw life after death.

After reading that article I started paying more attention to my friends who believed in that stuff. I listened to our publisher talk about souls, where they went, what she believed. I listened to stories about having guardian angels. In fact, our publisher told me during a car ride that I had two guardian angels. I felt my heart opening just a little to this idea of really believing in life after death, and, even more surprising to myself, unconventional thoughts about the universe behind this life.

During Thanksgiving weekend in 2009, our family got together with grandparents, aunts, uncles and cousins for a traditional family gathering. After our usual family ritual of playing dice in the hopes of winning a cup full of quarters, and calming the children who didn't win while stifling our own giggles, we started talking about spirituality. A friend had given me a crystal that was purely for spiritual purposes. The way the crystal was supposed to work was simple. As you held the crystal in one hand and dangled it above your other hand, you asked simple *yes* or *no* questions. If the answer was *yes*, it would gently swing in one direction; if the answer was *no*, it would swing the other way. Our entire family took turns, but I was the only one who seemed to take it seriously. I'll never forget Jesse holding the crystal in his hand, razzing me about my new found spiritual ideas.

The moment Jesse died I felt the *knowing* of him pass through me. I felt my heart and mind open up completely to the presence of Jesse beyond this life.

When everything happened I was so distraught I would have grasped at anything that offered me even five seconds of relief. The publisher of our magazine mentioned that she had run into our friend from the salon, and that she had offered me the opportunity to come in and talk to her. I couldn't wait. I felt there was a chance she could help me make the pain subside. I had expected the rest of my family to scoff at my intentions, but to my surprise, my 16-year-old daughter jumped at the chance to come with me.

We entered the salon having never met the woman featured in our magazine. She greeted us with the same smile that I had seen in the article. She took us back to her flow massage room and turned on some relaxing music. I was mesmerized, not just by the compassion she showed us, but because there seemed to be a glimpse of joy in her eyes, like she was about to tell us some good news – that she really believed my son was not only in a better place, but that his spirit was with us in that very room. I started sobbing.

We hoisted ourselves onto the massage table. I felt so much pain. It was unbearable, impossible to describe. There was this black hole that was left behind in my heart. She grabbed our hands and told us things about Jesse, about life after death, about what she felt, about what she knew. She told us that Jesse was in the room and that she had never seen such a funny kid. She belly-laughed in such a contagious way that I didn't know if I should laugh or cry. There were times when I did both simultaneously. She told us there would be times she wouldn't remember what she was saying, that Jesse would work through her. She told us that he was so happy, so full of energy and so very strong in his soul. She said he had already become stronger than most people who have been gone awhile. He was so excited to see us. She told me that he had indeed passed through me at the moment he died, as I had held his hand and wouldn't let go. I sobbed again as she said, "Oh, sweetie, don't you understand? He came through you to get to this world; he left through you too because he loved you most."

She told us to ask him questions. While we asked questions, there would be moments when Jesse would talk to her. He suggested that her music sucked and some Bob Marley was in order. She said she couldn't understand why he appeared to her as bald, constantly making something like a peace sign towards her. Later, we realized that this was the thumbs-up sign that he made all the time. But bald? His hair was his pride and joy. At the suggestion of the hospital staff, his dad and I had awkwardly cut off a piece of his hair while he lay dying. We wanted to have some small part of him. I should have known he wouldn't want us to touch that beautiful hair!

My first question came out in heaving sobs, "If I had stayed home that day, would you still be here? Would you have lived?" My friend smiled and said, "My dear Michelle, you were given a gift of this beautiful soul for 13 years, but he is no longer yours. He has bigger things to work on. What I feel from Jesse is that during his 13 years on earth he produced a resume of good – more than most people achieve in a lifetime and yet his work has barely begun." She then smiled towards Jesse and said, "He could have been sitting on your lap, Michelle. It wouldn't have mattered. It was his time, and now he is home." I remember wondering what that home was. I still haven't come up with an answer.

During our time in her office I kept leaning over from what I thought was my back straining. Eventually my friend said, "Can you feel that? He's pushing and leaning on you as hard as he can, trying to get you to notice him." As I cried, I felt him put his hand on my leg. I smiled. It was in that moment, as I stared at my friend, I noticed that her beautiful blue eyes were brown. For one of the happiest, most bittersweet moments of my life, I saw my little boy's beautiful brown eyes staring back at me. I was absolutely certain he was communicating these words, "I'm okay, mom. You'll be okay." No one will ever convince me otherwise.

Whatever works. That worked for me. You don't have to believe it, but I knew it to be true, and it helped.

During my meetings with her, I had so many wonderful moments with Jesse. Later, we noticed him in our dining room sitting at the table and sitting in the big chair in our living room. When I spoke to him in my car, he calmed my heart and hugged it in a way that's difficult to describe. He was present. I figured there would be a day when he would leave me, but for the time being, it helped me through my days. And I could tell it helped my other kids as well to be open to the idea of life after death. It helped them feel that they would see him again one day.

As I made my way through this new life, I was aware that there might be pitfalls. Anyone who knows me knows that I like to enjoy a glass of wine. Or a bottle. I won't deny it. I've been over-served at times, quite often by me. As people arrived at my house bearing pans of lasagna, they also brought cases of wine, which were well-received. I'm not proud to say it, but I drank too much wine at first. I would drown my brain at night. I had heard so many stories of other people who needed something to help them sleep at night. Knowing that others were sleeping at night while I lay wide awake drove me crazy. I couldn't cope with it at first. Drinking a few glasses of wine at night got me through. I know I shouldn't suggest that people drink to drown their sorrows, but that was my journey.

It reminded me of when my mom's husband died unexpectedly from a heart attack at the age of 49. I had been so proud of her for quitting smoking after my daughter was born. After years of kicking and screaming and begging her to stop smoking, she finally did. In the end, I don't think it was because of anything I said; it was her decision. When we received the news that her husband had died, the first thing

I handed her was a pack of cigarettes. Trying to take a breath those first few weeks was incredibly difficult. I didn't see it as the time to give up other vices.

The day came, however, when I said to myself, "Enough." I wasn't perfect. I fell back into my old ways every so often, but I was conscious of it. Sometimes, falling into the bottom of a bottle when feeling sad was the only way I could cope. In the end, I knew I had to be aware of my own vices, my own weaknesses. If I wasn't going to take care of myself, I realized I might need somebody to help me. Unfortunately, there were plenty of times when lying numb on the couch just pushed away the inevitable pain, and I had to feel the pain.

One of the things I caught myself doing, not only after Jesse's death but pretty much my entire life, was to throw myself at things. When my daughter started kindergarten, I was enthralled by the fact that the P.T.A. president's son was in her class. I thought for sure this would be my way into their little inner circle. I managed to get myself elected to the P.T.A. board. Within a year, I was the president of that board. Yep, that's me, full speed ahead. It was during my term as president of the P.T.A. that Jesse was diagnosed with type 1 diabetes. My perspective toward things that I and others had considered important quickly changed. At one meeting, I remember two parents arguing over whether or not we should share our new popcorn machine with a neighboring school. It was at that moment that I thought of my son and the obstacles we were facing. I thought to myself, "You know what? I have better things to do with my time than worry about a popcorn machine." I got up and walked out of that meeting, on to my next purpose.

In hindsight, it should come as no surprise that Jesse's diagnosis catapulted me into something meaningful as it related to his disease. Working with the diabetes community became my new passion. An idle body and mind always drove me crazy.

From the beginning, I was very open and public about Jesse's diabetes and very proud of my advocacy on his behalf and on behalf of others with this awful disease. After his death, I was inundated with emails and phone calls from around the world. I'm not trying to make it sound like I was so important, but I found that talking to others helped me through the first days and weeks after Jesse's death.

I will admit that diving into a new-found cause opened the doors to more responsibilities. As I wrote this, I was in the midst of planning Jessepalooza, a two-day rock festival in honor of Jesse. I had also been asked to help write a script for the upcoming Thunder Run Ride to Cure Diabetes, an event for which Jesse had been the ambassador the previous six years. Then, I did the voice-over for the script and talked about losing Jesse. Shortly after that, I got an email from a national TV show that I had appeared on to talk about Jesse being my inspiration for the Triabetes documentary. They wanted me to fly out and talk again about his loss and what I was doing now. I needed to take a DEEP. BREATH.

While all of this made me feel like I was doing something worthwhile to help keep Jesse's memory alive and to keep me from losing my mind, I quickly fell to pieces when something didn't go quite right. While planning Jessepalooza, we got a call that the venue had forgotten to put us down on their calendar and the dates had been given away. In my anger and frustration, I had a complete breakdown. I looked around and thought, "You did this to yourself, Michelle. You have no one to blame but yourself."

I knew I needed to give my brain a rest. I was an overcommitted disaster at this point. I didn't get overwhelmed easily, but at this point I was overwhelmed and exhausted.

Another thought that struck me was that I dreaded the idea of future events that I had promised to help with. For instance, each summer there was a large golf outing that would donate proceeds to JDRF. It was scheduled to take place seven months after Jesse's death.

I knew I needed to give my brain a rest. I was an overcommitted disaster at this point. I didn't get overwhelmed easily, but at this point I was overwhelmed and exhausted.

While many of the people I knew I would see there had already been through the grieving process with me, there would also be people there who had just learned of his death. The operative word here for me at that point was GUILT. I was worried I'd feel guilty if I smiled, guilty if I had a glass of wine, guilty if I chatted about something other than Jesse. It's how I felt. I didn't know how I would overcome those feelings.

I biked to work one morning. Usually I had to fight off thoughts of Jesse in order to maintain some kind of normalcy. As I biked that morning, my mind went once again to his moment of death. It occurred to me that I was grateful that the way he died was painless. He was unconscious, unknowing, unaware of his own passing. While dying has caused an amazing amount of grief for all of us, it caused Jesse no pain as it happened.

As these thoughts came to my mind I started crying again. What mother has to think thoughts like that? I actually had to let my brain go to "well at least he didn't suffer." I was distraught as I typed this. I felt physically ill when I thought about it. I suppose a lot of parents worry about their children being abducted, tortured, raped, brutalized, left to die. I was able to take some relief in knowing that Jesse didn't suffer and die painfully. I missed having plain old normal thoughts.

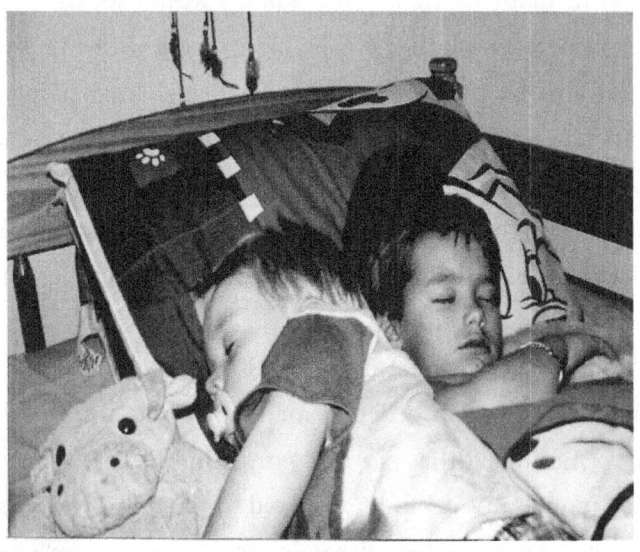

Jesse, age 5, with baby brother Joey
and much loved Moo Cow

4
Shopping at Target
(Two months after Jesse's death)

*"Only when we are no longer
afraid can we begin to live."
-Dorothy Thompson*

AFTER JESSE DIED, IT WAS A COUPLE OF weeks before I had any reason to venture out of the house to pick up supplies. After all, my house was inundated with well-meaning people who brought everything we needed, including those warm pans of lasagna.

I'll never forget my first trip to go shopping. It was hard to get up and get moving, but I knew it was time to get out there. I arrived at the store, took a deep breath and looked around hoping no one knew who I was. I was relieved to be there without a familiar person in sight who would no doubt say, "I'm so sorry for your loss." I didn't want to sound ungrateful. I felt like I'd be okay in a room full of anonymous people who didn't have a clue about the pain I was feeling.

I shopped for groceries at this store all the time and knew the aisles like the back of my hand. I could cruise through the aisles mindlessly, picking up the items that I needed.

It was a horrible thought to look around and feel so much pain and be so alone. I wanted everyone to feel the pain I was feeling.

As I was gliding along anonymously, my hand stopped short of the Crystal Light. So much pain and hurt flooded through me at that exact moment. It was the first time I realized I didn't need Crystal Light anymore. No one in my house had type 1 diabetes anymore. At that moment I burst into tears as memories and pain that I had pushed aside rushed back in. I picked up my cell phone and called Sandy, a friend of mine who has twin daughters with type 1 diabetes. I just needed someone – anyone – to talk to. I said, "Well, if you ever wondered what it would feel like the day diabetes left your life and your child left your life, this is it."

Then a different sort of pain set in as I watched other people shop. An old couple walked together and picked out groceries. A young mom with a happy, giggling two-year-old boy in her cart strolled past me. For as much as I wanted to remain unrecognized in the store, I looked around incredulously and thought, "How *dare* you not grieve for me?

Don't you know that my son *died*?" It was a horrible thought to look around and feel so much pain and be so alone. I wanted everyone to feel the pain I was feeling.

Then it occurred to me. As I stood there, a second thought hit me. Many of the people shopping that day were going through their lives mindlessly and full of pain, just like me. There was a mother who had lost a baby at birth, a grandmother who had lost a granddaughter. So much pain around me. It was like seeing that blue car again, the one I bought and thought no one else had before I started noticing them everywhere. Grief was no different; it was all around me. It was everywhere.

JESSE WAS HERE

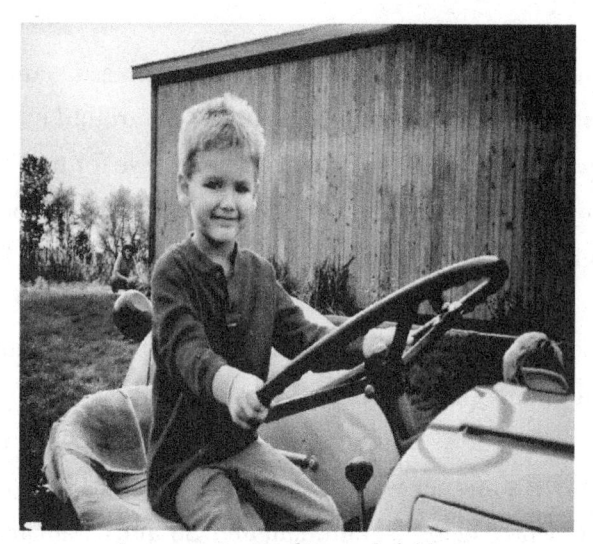

Jesse, age 5, pumpkin patch field trip

5
Dealing with the Dingleberries

(Three months after Jesse's death)

"There is nothing more beautiful than someone who goes out of their way to make life beautiful for others."
-Mandy Hale

DEATH IS SCARY, ESPECIALLY THE DEATH of a child. In our case, that feeling extended way beyond our immediate family and loved ones. It extended to everyone whose lives were touched.

A few days after Jesse's funeral, I felt it was important to have my other son return to his elementary school and try to assimilate with his new normal. Caring teachers and staff as well as sympathetic parents did their best to welcome him back. It broke my heart to watch him walk back through those doors, knowing he was forever changed.

One moment will stay with me forever. I pulled up to the school and noticed a neighbor boy who had grown up with my family standing with the safety patrol officer. He was crying. I realized he was crying because he had just seen my son. This sweet young man was utterly clueless as to what to say or do. His parents had made the decision to not only skip the funeral, but they also chose not to tell their two children what had happened. I couldn't read their minds or argue with their feelings of wanting to protect their children from learning about death so early in life. So, there stood that little boy on the sidewalk, trying to comprehend what he could already sense, that something bad had happened. He had heard the whispers but couldn't comprehend it in his little mind. For a second, I wanted to shake those parents, for by not telling their son what had happened to Jesse, it seemed to me they were doing more harm than good.

The fact was, I had to grow thicker skin.

There would also be pain as it related to the team from the endocrinology department that had seen Jesse battle type 1 diabetes since he was three years old. No other child in our area had died from this disease, so you can imagine how many parents were calling me, worried that this could happen to their children. It pained me to learn that the diabetes team that knew us personally was telling parents not to worry, that this would not happen to their children. What they didn't realize, as I now knew, they were doing a disservice to these families because people, indeed children, could die from type 1 diabetes. By telling other families it couldn't happen to them made me feel like they were dismissing my family as though we had done something wrong in managing his disease. It seemed cruel and unfair.

The fact was, I had to grow thicker skin. Later on, I read so much misinformation on the Internet about what had happened to my son, but most of it was speculation and gossip. I could have lashed out; I wanted to scream at all of them. Instead, I dug deep to find the grace and dignity to know and understand that we did everything we could for Jesse. I let them gossip. I stayed strong and true for myself and my family. It's all I could do.

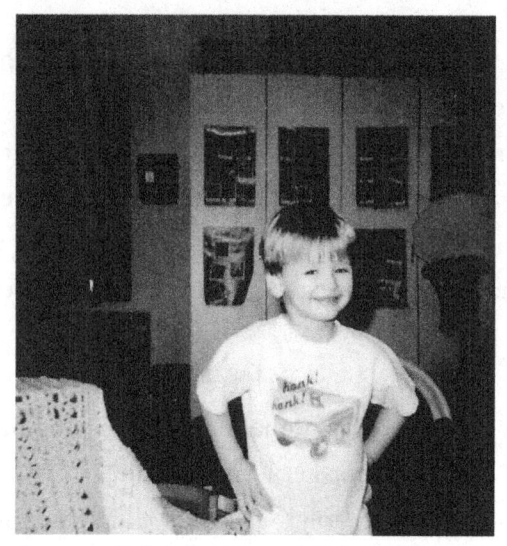

Jesse, age 3, first day of type 1 diabetes diagnosis
March 3, 2000

6
Everyone Grieves Differently

(Four months after Jesse's death)

> *"Where you used to be, there is a hole in the world, which I find myself constantly walking around in the daytime, and falling in at night. I miss you like hell."*
> -Edna St. Vincent Millay

YES, IT'S TRUE. EVERYONE GRIEVES DIFFERently. One night our family went to my 10-year-old's Little League game. Not unusual for our family although this was his first year in Little League. In past years, we had gone to watch Jesse play. The Little League park was alive with reminders of Jesse, particularly when we saw a lot of the same families that we used to hang out with. Since this was the first game we had attended since Jesse's death, I wondered how I would feel walking through the park, people smiling and laughing and chatting with me. I sensed it was actually more difficult for my 16-year-old daughter than for me.

My daughter grieved differently than I did. While we are very similar in the way we manage our feelings – a little pushy, a little bossy – when it came to Jesse's death, we handled our emotions very differently. My daughter showed a lot of anger. She got angry at people who tried to memorialize Jesse through social media sites or by creating t-shirts or hats with sayings about him or even participating in the rock festival we had planned to host. She wanted everyone to grieve the way she grieved, but that's just not the way it works. She had her processes; I had mine.

While walking to the diamond where my son played, we ran into the mother of one of Jesse's best friends. He was like family. While the mom and I were talking about the boys as they played in the field, I could tell my daughter was angry because her answers were short and curt. While I chatted with his mom about how things were going, my daughter started talking about how much she hated when people that she didn't even know would come up to her and tell her how sorry they were. She said, "I just want them to stay away. I don't know them, and I don't care how they feel." I tried explaining to her that those people meant well and maybe didn't have the right words to say. To her, at this point, the right words would have been no words at all.

As I wrote this four months after Jesse's death, I still had not gone to any formal grief counseling. I knew at some point I might need it. Right after Jesse's death, I did go online and look up grief counseling. I ended up getting lost in a sea of websites from all over the world. There was a local grief group in my city, but as I read about it, one thing became clear to me early on – I had no desire to sit in a room with a mother who lost her son to a suicide, or a daughter who's mom died after a long battle with cancer. I didn't mean to sound harsh or uncaring, but I knew it would be difficult for me to try and grieve with other people who were not walking in my shoes, who had not experienced the exact same grief as me.

Case in point, about one month after my world went to hell, my friends were hosting a costume party at their beautiful home. I wasn't exactly ready to go out in public. After all, I wasn't quite sure yet how I would answer questions like "How many kids do you have?" or "How old are your kids?" Who wants to go to a party as Debbie Downer? I sure didn't. Still, I wanted everyone on earth to know about my amazing son, that we hadn't forgotten him, that we wanted to be recognized as going through something horrible.

I sucked it up. I responded to the invitation because she

was one of my best friends who had helped me through the worst of my days. I knew she would be careful to prep people before I arrived.

Upon our arrival, we quickly dipped into the margaritas, donned our beads and masks and started chatting. Damn, it felt GOOD! It felt GOOD to be talking about something other than Jesse. I was still filled with sadness, but for a moment or two I felt like a normal human being again. We talked with new and different people and I discovered that it felt good that they didn't know what had happened to us. My friend then introduced me to a very nice lady who had recently lost her 20-year-old son unexpectedly. It had been over a year since his death and she had clearly not moved forward, not even an inch. I would never criticize people for how they grieved, but this woman clearly had not found any solace over the past year. She was so sad. I quickly realized we would not relate and would never be close friends. I could tell instantly that my grieving was very different than hers. I knew that constant, never-ending grieving would suck me into an abyss of depression and alcohol, conditions under which I could not live. Her grief was like poison to me. I realized she would find comfort by seeking out others who were feeling and grieving the same way she was. She'd find her way; I just knew my way would be different.

As the evening progressed, I ran into a wonderful man

who had done a lot of charity work for the diabetes community. He was a fireman with a big heart – that was clear. Then he asked the question I had been dreading. "So, how is your son with diabetes doing?"

I had to say, "My son died a month ago." Ugh. The world's biggest ugh. Pain again. But as we talked, his sympathetic ear really helped me. Moments later his drunk girlfriend came up and didn't know what we had been talking about. He was talking to my friends and me about a diabetes fundraiser. She got this look of distaste on her face and said, "Oh, I don't know if we are going to that. I can't keep all of these charity things straight." I'm confident in saying that she was less than comfortable with the barrage of friends who came to my rescue and almost threw her to the ground in anger. I'm guessing she learned a quick lesson about awareness and sensitivity as four of my friends chastised her for her callous behavior. I realized she most likely meant no harm, but I'm guessing she walked away with a new sense of how to interject herself into a new conversation.

The entire evening helped me realize I needed to seek out people who had gone through what I was living, who could really FEEL what I was feeling.

I found myself grieving with others via social media. I had always spent quite a bit of time on social media. I found it helpful to be able to stay in touch with pretty much anybody on the planet. I'll never forget having to tell my friend to post on my social media accounts that Jesse had died. It felt so crass – so harsh – yet, I have to say, it was one of the best things I could have done. It got the message out quickly without me having to try to get through phone conversations with a thousand different people. It allowed me to grieve in a public forum.

One message I got was from a man named Bryan, whom I had gone to high school with years before. He now lived on the West Coast and, aside from social media, I'll admit I probably wouldn't have recognized him anymore. He posted immediately after Jesse's death, "Amy (his wife) and I are heartbroken and can't imagine the pain you are feeling. We pray for you every day."

One week to the day after Bryan posted that on my account, I saw this on Bryan's social media, "I have lost the love of my life tonight. Amy died in a car crash. I am lost." He had been left with four children – one who was just learning to walk – so he also turned to social media to reach out to people. While Bryan and I were not grieving the same loss, what we were doing was grieving at the same time and feeling each other's pain with burning reality. We helped each other as we moved along, checking in and knowing that when we would say to each other "I'm thinking of you," we really meant it.

In the same breath, I can also say that posting status

updates about how I was feeling was like cutting into my arm and feeling the relief of bleeding. It was a strange feeling of painful cleansing. Each thought I poured into my updates helped me heal just a little. It was helpful because I knew my friends and family could keep tabs on me. They all knew when I was feeling hopeless (and needed a big pan of lasagna with a bottle of Cabernet!) or when I was actually doing okay. It saved me from a thousand incoming calls and also gave me a sense of relief that by posting my thoughts I always had someone to talk to.

Through social media I had already met a lot of people and had stayed connected to many people I had met in the diabetes world. When the news of Jesse's death started spreading, I found myself being a magnet for other people who had lost children to this disease – real live human beings who were sharing my little corner of hell. I know it sounds strange, but I considered this to be a true gift. I desperately wanted to talk to others who could relate to what I was going through.

Sadly, two weeks later, my wish came true. I saw a post on a friend's social media account that a young man named Trent had died unexpectedly at the age of 14. He had been diagnosed with type 1 diabetes three days before Jesse. He had died in the middle of the night from a low blood sugar event. I had never heard of this family, but man, I was drawn to talk to them. I got a call from Tom, a friend in the diabetes world, asking if he could connect us. I anxiously agreed. I just needed to hear them, feel them and say, "I know how you're feeling."

My first correspondence was an email to Jen, his mother. At the time, she was too grief-stricken to talk on the phone, which I understood completely. Her son had died on a Thursday morning. Jen was an E.R. nurse blessed with an amazing husband and three beautiful children. She was walking proof that, yes, bad things happened to good families. I felt an immediate sisterhood with this woman. My heart ached for her because I knew her every thought and move – staring at the bedroom, the guilt of thinking she could have prevented his death somehow, not knowing how to help her kids deal with it, not being able to stop her husband from crying. I knew it; I felt it; I lived it.

I stood by her side figuratively. They had to wait for an autopsy before they could finalize funeral plans. The funeral had to be delayed over a week but ended up being held on Easter Sunday, a fortuitous day for that Christian family.

At the same time, I found myself talking to two other amazing moms in Florida who had each lost children, ages 22 and 23, to type 1 diabetes. They had lost their children two years ago and four years ago, respectively. The moms, Sara and Laurie, had given me a glimpse of my future. I'll be honest, while it appeared tolerable, it was a reality check that my pain wasn't going anywhere anytime soon. I knew certain feelings would be coming back when least expected. That the visual of an ambulance driving by would always make me think, "Those cars need to move over! That could be my son!" That birthdays and Mother's Day would hurt. That pain was going to park itself on my doormat for years to come. But, wow! How wonderful it was to have these sisters to email and call.

The entire evening helped me realize I needed to seek out people who had gone through what I was living, who could really FEEL what I was feeling.

As the months passed, I found myself texting Jen when I heard a song that reminded me of Jesse. I'd call her to share a laugh. We'd share smiles and toasts by our pools while we chatted on video calls. We would cry together when we couldn't seem to help pulling out one of our son's skateboards and hugging it tightly to our bodies. It made our craziness seem okay.

In the same respect, I found that same kind of friend-based grief counseling to be helpful for my children. Jen and Bob had children that could relate to my children.

They could feel guilty together, feel sad together and share when they had a good day. What a wonderful world we live in when we can find people to grieve with us during difficult times.

It's good to know there are pans of warm lasagna being prepared all over the world just waiting to be shared.

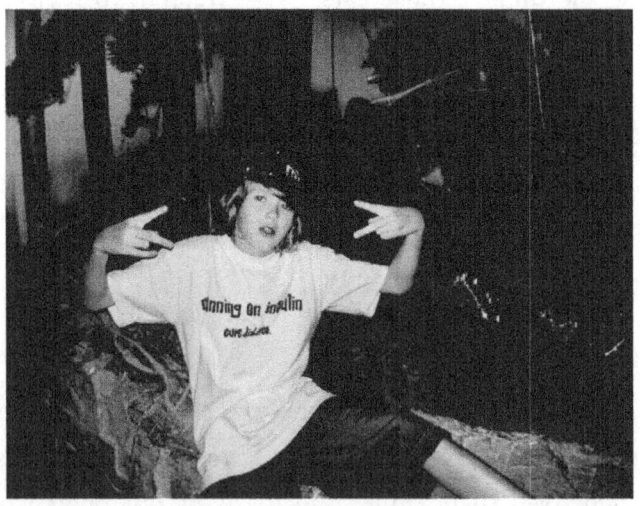

Jesse, age 13, last family trip, just months before he died

7
Turning a Corner

(Four months after Jesse's death)

> *"I don't understand why you
> have to go through
> the dark to see the light."*
> -Anna Eager

YOU ARE GOING TO HAVE BAD DAYS. THAT'S the reality. There's nothing you can do about it, and nothing your friends and family can help you with. That's how I was feeling as I wrote this on the worst day I had since the initial shock of Jesse's death. I wanted to share this while I was feeling that way so I wouldn't forget the sheer pain of the day.

It all started the night before. I had been angry with my 16-year-old daughter for her unwillingness to allow Jesse to be a "poster child" (her words) for diabetes. I had always wanted her to be part of the world of diabetes advocacy with me, but that wasn't her role in Jesse's life. Her role was to be Jesse's confidante and sounding board, the person he could turn to and talk about things that he hated at times – his teachers, his school and me. Most importantly, he needed somebody to talk to about his diabetes, and I was not that person.

I was also upset with her because at one point she had agreed to go to group grief counseling at Hospice with her younger brother, and now she was refusing to go. I was feeling pressure from the outside world. Should I force her to go? Does she really need it? She was a lot like me and there were times when I felt the same way about counseling.

After a nice dinner the whole family rolled up their sleeves to tackle painting a portion of our swimming pool. (I realize this sounds awful, but it was a nice let's-work-together-as-a-family moment.) We finished up at nightfall and thought it would be fun to sit around our firepit in the backyard with some friends. Later, after our friends left, my daughter and I found ourselves talking about Jesse. For months, my daughter and I had held our feelings in. Now, with a glass of wine in my hand, I was finally able to talk to her about that awful day. Every detail. What she was feeling, what I was feeling, the horrible feelings of guilt we had about that day. Could we have prevented it? Would he be here if we had acted differently? We also talked about the beautiful moments we spent together with him in the hospital room as he neared death. We talked about how we could hardly believe it was him in that bed. We shared our feelings about how we still felt his presence.

My daughter finally went to bed at 1:00 a.m. Instead of going to bed, I watched videos of Jesse and cried for hours. I cried so much that when I woke up the next morning my eyes were so swollen I was embarrassed to show up at my son's school for a presentation. I found myself in such a funk that I didn't want to get out of bed. I worked from home and dragged myself to a lunch date I had made earlier. I figured, "What the hell? My day already sucks, I might as well continue the torture and go to school to pick up Jesse's yearbook and his artwork." And so I did.

I walked over to the school and into the office. Thankfully, nobody in the hallway knew me or recognized me. I asked the school secretary for Jesse's belongings and she graciously handed them to me without saying much. I clutched the world's ugliest handmade coffee mug that Jesse had made in art class as if it was a Picasso, sobbing the whole way to the car. Four hours later I was still mentally exhausted from just 'being.' I knew there was still a lot of 'doing' left for me.

Toward the end of the school year I did receive a brief note from one of his teachers:

JESSE WAS HERE

> Hi Michelle,
>
> We set up the new display case with Jesse's plaque and some other things, so the rest of his items are in the main office for you to pick up. There is also a yearbook for you. Page 21 is dedicated to Jesse.
>
> I hope you're doing well, :)
>
> Kris

The emotions I felt were terrible sadness and anger. It had been just over three months since Jesse died. The idea of trudging into his school made me feel so sad. I should have been feeling proud that the kids had dedicated a whole page in the yearbook to my son, but all I felt was sadness and emptiness. I was thinking about the fact that his entire adulthood was stolen from him, that this would be the last time his smiling face would be in a yearbook. I knew the yearbook would be something I'd go back to and look at over the years just to feel close to him. Even worse, the kids would always remember him as the kid who died when they were young.

When I was in 5th grade, a boy in 8th grade who lived down the street attempted to swim across a pond and drowned. I remembered it very well even though I wasn't a close friend. After 30 years, when I visited my hometown, I still stared at his house when I drove by. "There's the house of John Faanes; it's so sad that he died so young." Now my son would be the John Faanes for these kids. They would think sad thoughts about him for the rest of their lives.

In the end, I chose to go and pick up the yearbook. I walked in quietly and asked for his things. Two days later I thought "Why not leave the yearbook there for the kids to sign one last time?" I gave the book back to one of his best friends and received many grateful messages from the kids. They thanked me for the opportunity to once again share how they were feeling.

I was surprised that I was able to speak with ease during the interview, choking back tears only twice. I think it was because I felt so much amazing support from the others in the room. I felt connected once again to this disease – and to my son.

It was at this point in time that I was asked to tell my story on national television.

Two months after Jesse died I got a message from the

producers of a television show on CNBC called "dLife." I had been on the show during happier times when I had produced a documentary about 12 type 1 athletes who were training for an Ironman distance triathlon. During that initial segment, I was beaming when I talked about this work. I told the audience how Jesse had inspired all of it. He didn't just inspire me, he inspired all these other athletes that were training for a life changing event.

This time the producers asked me to come on the show and tell Jesse's story – to talk about his death and how I was able to move forward. Though I agreed to fly out and do the segment, I questioned myself and how I might appear to others. Would others realize that I continued to do this sort of thing in an effort to help others? Would they realize that this type of work helped me to keep going? That it gave my life – and Jesse's death – some sense of purpose? That I still craved to be part of this community that I threw myself at when Jesse was diagnosed? All of those questions went through my head.

With plenty of doubts in my mind, I booked my flight still wondering what I would talk about or if I could even get through the interview. When I arrived on set, I was immediately surrounded by people from the diabetes community. I knew I had made the right choice. No one was judging me because of the fact that it had only been four months since

Jesse died. Instead, they spoke about the courage it must have taken for me to come forward.

I was surprised that I was able to speak with ease during the interview, choking back tears only twice. I think it was because I felt so much amazing support from the others in the room. I felt connected once again to this disease – and to my son. Although, I have to admit, I couldn't turn around and look at the photos of my son that were flashing on the screen behind me. That would have been too much to bear.

The segment was filmed in a room with 35 people present. Throughout the interview, I felt this intense feeling of pride. The strangest sensation I had was one of feeling like I was home. I was home with these people and I was so grateful – grateful to be allowed to talk about my son and continue to let his life have value. I don't know how else to explain that overwhelming feeling of gratitude.

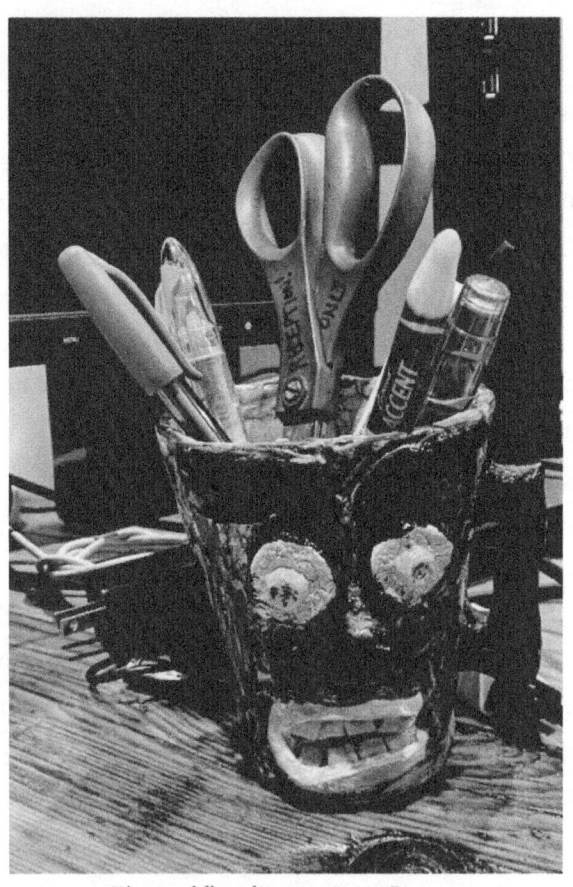

The world's ugliest mug, my Picasso

8
Since Everything Happened

(Five months after Jesse's death)

"We are healed of a suffering only by experiencing it to the fullest."
-Marcel Proust

WHEN JESSE WAS DIAGNOSED WITH diabetes, I noticed that my entire family did something peculiar. When we would look at family photos or talk about memories we would all catch ourselves saying, "Oh, remember? That was before Jesse had diabetes." Whether it was his cute, smiling face in his two-year-old photo or talking about the time we went to the fireworks together, someone would inevitably say, "Oh, yeah, that was before Jesse got diabetes."

A few days after I noticed it was exactly five months since Jesse died, I went to grab a drink with an old friend. She and I were thick as thieves since high school, into our marriages and after the birth of our respective three kids. The last time we had really connected was when her youngest daughter was born and she made Jesse's dad and me the godparents. Time and distance caused a disconnect, so when Jesse died, I realized I didn't even have her phone number anymore.

She found me nonetheless. I was excited to get a message from her that she had an appointment in town and would like to get together. In the midst of catching up on our families and our lives, I caught myself saying repeatedly, "Since everything happened." I'd say things like, "Well, thanks, but I've gained 20 pounds since everything happened." Or, "The kids have been doing pretty well since everything happened." And the craziest thing of all, "Jesse's dad and I have been getting along so much better since everything happened."

Somewhere in the five months since Jesse died, I stopped referring to my son's death as, "When Jesse died." Instead, it became, "Since everything happened." I'm not sure why. It's not hard to say, "When Jesse died." It's just that I worried sometimes about the people I was talking to. I worried that it had been five months and they might be tired of me going on and on about my life, my pain, my bad days, my good days – just all of it.

I also caught myself using another phrase quite often: "Well, except for the funeral." I found myself in so many conversations with friends or family talking about someone else. Since I hadn't had a chance to talk to anyone for very long that day, I found myself saying, "The last time I talked to Carl was at the gala. Well, except for the funeral."

Jen, the mother of Trent, the 14-year-old who had died just a few weeks after Jesse, noticed that she found herself always saying, "When our lives fell apart."

Both phrases were clearly for those of us suffering through the first few months after losing a child.

For the previous five years, Jesse had been Junior Ambassador for a diabetes-related event called Thunder Run. During those years we filmed commercials for the event and participated in it with another family, whose son Aaron was diagnosed about the same time as Jesse. Our families remained close over the years while his dad and I served on the board of JDRF. His mom and I rode our bikes through Death Valley together in honor of our boys.

Thunder Run was always Jesse's favorite event. He didn't like being a poster child for his disease, but he didn't mind speaking to the Harley Davidson owners about the event. He ate up the attention while he proudly climbed on the back of his dad's Hog each year at the front of the pack with the officers who lead the ride.

After Jesse's death we struggled with what our participation should be in the event going forward. I had always served on the committee that wrote the script and filmed the commercial. They politely asked me again if I would be willing to not only help write it, but to be in the commercial with my kids, with Jesse as the focus. I agreed and carefully wrote the script to not sound like we were lost. I wanted to sound hopeful for others. So we talked about how relentless a disease diabetes was and then talked about how we were going to be just as relentless in the fight to find a cure for others.

The time for Thunder Run arrived quickly. I was excited that family members who lived a few hours away were coming down for the event. It would bring together a lot of people that I knew and loved. However, when morning came, I found myself getting weepy while getting ready. Since the kids were riding with their dad and my partner, I was off on my own in the car to drive 30 minutes to the event.

After a few minutes alone in the car, not really understanding why I was so upset, I burst into tears. Of course I knew why I was upset. I was going to be seeing people who knew and loved Jesse. I knew they would all be feeling sorry for me. The pain was going to be strong that day and I had set myself up for it, hadn't I?

I pulled into the parking lot still talking out loud to Jesse, asking him to please help me get through the day. I wiped away the tears, put on my strong face and marched out. The first person I saw was my sister and her adorable eight-year-old son. He was standing there grinning like a fool, and I quickly came up to give him a hug. Then, I saw he was wearing a Walk to Cure Diabetes t-shirt that I had created in 2001. It said "Jesse got Diabetes and All I Got was this Lousy T-shirt!" On his head he was wearing a bandana that said, "It's better to burn out than to fade away. Jesse T. Alswager 1996-2010." I had completely forgotten that the Hog chapter had made bandanas in his memory. As I choked back tears, I started to feel sick to my stomach. I looked around in disbelief but with a tremendous amount of pride as I saw the bandanas everywhere – on the tops of riders' heads, tied around arms and necks and even on one of the on-duty police officers. I donned my sunglasses and quietly cried to myself. I could tell people noticed and felt terrible for me.

I decided I needed to pull myself together – again. I knew this was a "five months later" reaction because I honestly didn't want others to feel bad. I walked up to a gentleman who had just lost his best friend two weeks before. He was an amazing man who deserves mention in this book. He was a kind, gentle man who gave thousands of dollars to diabetes research, specifically in Jesse's honor that particular year.

The last time I had seen him was at Jesse's funeral. I went to offer my condolences because, who better than me to say,

"I know how you feel." We cried together and carried each other's pain, It felt SO good to be able to help him deal with the loss of his best friend.

After being interviewed by the news crew as my peppy-imaged alter-ego, I turned around and saw Jesse's face looking right at me with his now-famous "thumbs up" image. The flag they put on the back of the lead motorcycle as a tribute to Jesse was being photographed with me and everyone else. It was time to ride. It was a bittersweet moment getting on a motorcycle and not being able to look back and see Jesse riding with his dad, who always rode next to Aaron, his partner in crime. At the same time, I started to grin through my tears at the sight of Jesse's siblings riding proudly for him.

As the day went on I found myself being able to smile and enjoy the company of many people I hadn't seen in a while. Then came the moment where Aaron went on stage with Cody, a five-year-old boy who had been diagnosed with type 1 diabetes at the age of 13 months. I had greeted Cody in my office the day he was diagnosed. The cutest little boy ever was now standing on the stage as Aaron introduced him as the new ambassador for Thunder Run. I put my sunglasses back on, fought the pain and watched through tears as my son was replaced.

I'm a reasonable person. I understood that Jesse could never be replaced. I also understood that the world was moving forward. Still, the pain I felt at that moment was excruciating and I wanted it to be over as quickly as possible.

The evening came to an end. My family and I, along with Jesse's dad, returned to our home to sit by the pool and the firepit, share some happy memories and talk about good times. Jesse's dad and I took a few moments to reflect on how nice it had been that we got along and could support each other through this whole tragic ordeal.

I woke up the next day to have breakfast with our visiting relatives but couldn't shake the funk and found myself back in bed for a long nap. I learned that whenever we did something in Jesse's honor, anything intense, we could anticipate a couple of days' worth of pain and sadness. While it always felt good to honor him, there was pain that accompanied the memories.

What I started to understand about myself was that the ebb and flow of grief seemed to be a two-day ordeal. If we did something to honor Jesse, the second day was when the sadness seemed to hit the hardest. I don't have answers as to why that happened, but I noticed it in my entire family. The second night after Thunder Run, I noticed myself still feeling pretty sad. I especially noticed that my youngest son, who had been very resilient, was still upset as well. So, I scheduled myself to work from home the next day in order to be present for him. I even suggested he invite some friends over to swim. I fell asleep after making those arrangements and had my second horrible dream about Jesse.

I knew from experience that a lot of my friends had experienced terrible dreams about the people they had lost. I hadn't, to this point. This was only my second dream about Jesse, but both were disturbing. In this dream – what I can remember of it – Jesse was wearing his little glasses from when he was younger. He was telling me that he didn't have much time and that he was going to die. Even though the images in my dream were different than the actual moments before he died, in many ways the dream played out the same, except that Jesse was conscious and was telling me the next steps, almost guiding me through his death. He was so much younger in the dream. We just snuggled and allowed death to take him once again, without me having any choice. I woke up with vivid memories of those thoughts and, very much like the day he died, I forced myself to shut those thoughts off. Five months later, it was still raw and painful.

Five months after Jessed died was also the first time I really started noticing a disconnect between me and my family and friends.

I was sitting with a group of friends who were helping me plan a big rock festival in Jesse's memory. These people were all good friends who cared about me and loved me, my family and Jesse. We were scrambling to get the music lined up, the prizes organized and the volunteers committed when a comment was made, "Well, next year I just look forward to having more time to plan this." Immediately after the words left my friend's mouth, she knew it was an awful thing to say. I said, "He died five months ago." The reality of the moment was that even though she was close to me and held his hand in the hospital as he died, she had taken a larger leap away from that awful day than I had. I couldn't really blame her; I just knew it to be her reality.

The reality for me was that just hours ago I was sorting laundry into piles on my bed as I always did. I pulled a t-shirt out of the pile that said "I'll Gladly Trade My Sister." Without any hesitation I thought, "Does this go in Jesse's pile or Joey's?" It made me take a deep breath, and I remembered that it hadn't been that long since I had lost Jesse. I was nowhere near where others were in the grieving process.

Flashbacks are a real thing. I was cruising along pretty good as far as the grieving world goes (yeah, I've actually thought of it in those terms), writing this book, creating big events in my son's name and returning to work full throttle. Sure, I noticed some bumps in the road, like sobbing all the way to work or breaking down when a client that I hadn't talked to in a few months found out what happened and I had to go back to square one to deal with the pain. All in all, on a scale of 1-10, I would have given myself a resounding eight in the "dealing with it" department.

After the unexpected death of my friend's baby girl, a baby I had never met, the flashbacks and dreams began.

Over those few months when I thought of Jesse, I couldn't think happy thoughts or shut out the feelings that hurt or caused immediate pain. After the start of the first beautiful dream I had about Jesse, what followed caused me a great deal of pain. I was becoming concerned for my own well-being.

After a few days of pool time with the kids and visits from lots of friends, we settled back into our normal routine. I had my first good dream about Jesse. Up to this point, I had dreamed two dreams about Jesse and both of them were horrifying. They left me sad and it took days to recover. This new dream was different. It wasn't like Jesse came to me to tell me something profound or point to God and say, "Hey, mom, how cool is this dude, yo?" No, it was more like he was part of the family, enjoying us again as one big group. What stands out most to me about this dream is that I didn't wake up sad. When I woke up, I remembered seeing his big, beautiful brown eyes in the dream.

Jesse had an eye disorder that most people didn't know about. He could not look to the left with his left eye because of some nerve issues, another wonderful physical disorder given to my beautiful son. Never one to feel sorry for himself, once in a while he would purposefully make his eyes go crossed just to tick me off. He knew it irked me.

In this dream I kept commenting on how wonderful it was to look into those brown eyes. I can remember actually being able to feel him in this dream. He was there. I was grateful to have a happy thought of him, even though it was in my subconscious state. But, true to form, Jesse couldn't just let it go at that. No, he had to go cross-eyed and wait for me to chastise him before he'd giggle his sweet little laugh. I woke up with a strange sense of satisfaction, even happiness.

> *For the rest of my life I will never forget a firefighter who looked at me and, with a strong handshake that turned into a hug, said, "I'm Lorenzo. I worked on your son."*

Still, as the days passed by I noticed another ugly slideshow bubbling to the surface. The flashbacks I was having were actually starting to scare me. For instance, I kept hearing his dad on the phone saying, "He's not breathing!" and then me screaming, "NO!" I didn't understand why this was happening. I tried to shut it off, but it was like my brain was saying, "Nope, today you're going to deal with this whether you like it or not."

Five months in, I just wanted to get back to being my normal go-getter self and not deal with the pain. I kept asking myself if I was really ready. I knew that if these awful slideshows kept popping up, I would finally have to go talk to somebody. I was not looking forward to that because I knew this tuna can had some jagged edges that would cut me pretty damn deep.

It was at this moment in time that I decided to go visit the fire station that had gotten the call to my house on that fateful day.

On the day of Jesse's death, I walked up to my house. It was filled with police officers, detectives and firefighters. In addition, there were others present who were already getting ready to transport my son to the hospital in hopes of reviving him.

I was not kind to the first responders that day. I spewed at them and nearly took off the head of a detective who said "Oh, he has a pulse! Michelle, that is such a good thing!"

I screamed, "Are you fucking kidding me? It's been more than 40 minutes! He's DEAD!" I don't actually remember saying those things – I'm told I did. I was in shock.

Despite what happened that day, many of the first responders, even the attending physician at the hospital, streamed into the funeral, so sad and so kind. The doctor just shook his head in disbelief as if he could still not fathom what happened to this young man.

Weeks later the same detective that I had screamed at, stopped by my house for the dreaded visit. She was delivering the death belongings – Jesse's pants, phone, glucose meter, etc. I hugged the bag while she talked to me and asked how I was doing. I could tell she was uncomfortable. At the time, I admitted to her that I was doing shitty. She talked to me about how hard that day was on all of them, how they had all been following me and my family since it happened and couldn't get us out of their minds.

In response, I did something that I thought would be cathartic for them and me. I invited them to our big Jessepalooza rock festival. I even stopped by their stations to drop off posters. I went in feeling brave and promised myself I wouldn't cry. I rang the buzzer at the first stop, and the firefighter who answered the door said, "You're Jesse's mom." I told them about the event and explained that I wanted to invite them because I thought it was important for them to see that we were doing okay. That, even though they saw us on the worst day of our lives, we wanted them to know that we understood how hard they tried to help Jesse. I also wanted them to know that we all had to move forward and still show love for each other.

For the rest of my life I will never forget a firefighter who looked at me, and with a strong handshake that turned into a hug he said, "I'm Lorenzo. I worked on your son." I cried.

I couldn't help it. He was clearly hurt by the events of that day, and it felt damn good for me to tell them to come and enjoy Jessepalooza and see that we were doing our level best to survive.

The same went for the detective I verbally attacked. When I told her about the event, she was ecstatic. They were all happy to be included and said they would be there.

I found that by reaching out to them, it was cleansing to me to be able to bring some sort of good back into their lives. While they didn't save my Jesse, they sure as hell tried. Each of them had to go back to their families and try to forget what had happened.

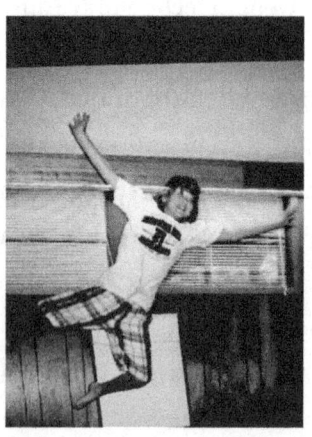

Jesse, 13, jumping on the bed

MICHELLE BAUER

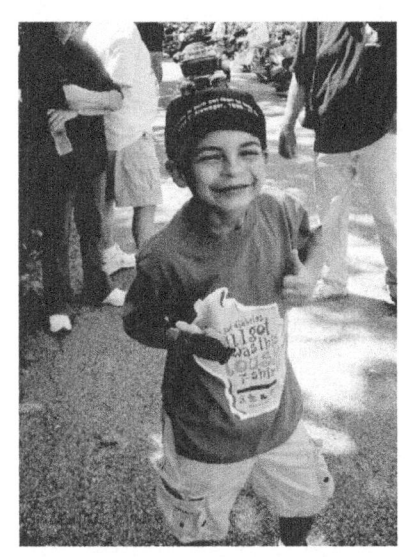

Mason, Jesse's cousin, at Thunder Run

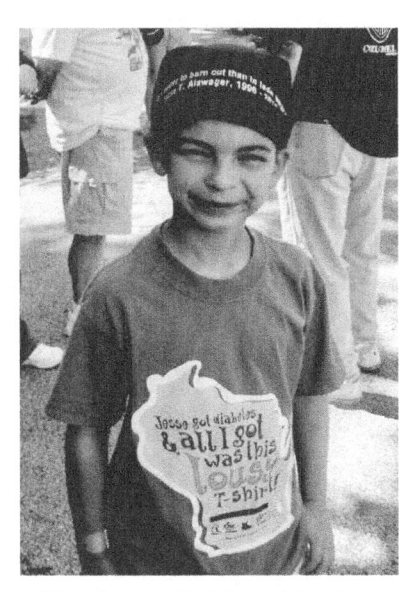

Thunder Run T-shirt and bandana

9
An Ambulance is Just an Ambulance

(Six months after Jesse's death)

> *"It isn't for the moment you are struck that you need courage, but for the long, uphill climb back to sanity and faith and security."*
> -Anne Morrow Lindbergh

SO THERE WE WERE. MONTH SIX. NO pomp and circumstance, just another date we tracked as we moved forward. I'm sure I'm not terribly different from any other parent who has lost a child. The moment everything happened was the worst day of my life. Anne Morrow Lindbergh's words resonated for me personally because it's true that the courage I needed that day paled in comparison to what I needed to endure as time moved on.

I thought about many things as I tried to find the best way to express myself to others, especially as I wrote this book.

One thing I had read in other books dealing with grief was that I might experience short-term memory loss. I was grateful, actually, when I read that was a symptom of grief. I could run a major event but couldn't remember that five minutes ago I had told Joey I would take him to his baseball game and then forgot to do it. I noticed those closest to me started becoming annoyed by this. It was frustrating for me, but I told them I couldn't help it and that lashing out didn't help me in return. I didn't forget things because I was trying to be sloppy or irritating; I forgot things because that is how my brain was working those days and I could only hope my memory would return as I healed.

At six months, I found myself arguing more with my teenage daughter. While she was a great kid, she tended to focus on her anger and took it out on those closest to her. I found over those first six months I was too easy on her – partly because I was thinking about all she had been through, partly because I just didn't have the energy to care at times. That's the honest truth. I mean, who gives a rip about a soda can being left out when my son had just died? I didn't care. The pressure from the outside sometimes became so strong that I had to change my thinking. Maybe that's what tough love is all about. I finally felt strong enough to tell my daughter that her words were hurting me, that I couldn't take that kind of energy thrown my way any longer.

I knew it would be tough for her as I changed the rules back to normal and set higher expectations for her behavior, her grades and her respect for me. I offered to get her counseling and, while she had been on the verge of accepting that help, she always retreated. As any parent knows, not all parental decisions are good ones. What I learned as I grew as a parent was that sometimes decisions just needed to be made.

Later we would learn if those decisions were the right ones. That was how I felt about the decision not to force my kids into counseling. I was hopeful that I wouldn't regret that decision someday.

As for my relationship at home, I wrote earlier about what a struggle it had become to be intimate. The idea of experiencing joy or feeling good was unacceptable to me. I truly believed in the beginning that I would never find joy again or experience another intimate relationship. But the reality is that I did find joy again.

From the beginning, there were a lot of emotional hurdles in my relationship that I had to face. I found myself in a lot of arguments, mostly because that relationship was no longer the number one priority in my life. The relationship with my significant other at the time was not healthy before Jesse's death and I knew it.

After experiencing the grief of Jesse's death, I found other things in my life trivial, some not worth fixing. I'm not saying that was the right attitude to have, but it was my reality at the time.

The best advice I could give anyone trying to manage a relationship after a tragedy like this is simple: BE PATIENT. I can honestly say that I didn't have the energy to fix anything at that time. My love life just wasn't that important to me. Would it be in six months? Perhaps. But being pushed and pushed wasn't helping me at all and only made both of us more frustrated.

I had to let some things go and not make a big deal out of some small things, and still I found myself at the point of not even being close to being healed.

If you see this happening to others in similar situations, I can only emphasize patience. Patience is the key.

At one point I had a business meeting with a wonderful client. When I first met her I thought she was quite important in our community because she knew a lot of people. My previous boss (who owned the same company) had talked a lot about her over the years. Suffice it to say, I was intimidated when I met her. The first time she and I sat down, the company I worked for had shut down for three months while a new owner came on board to start the business back up. I was struggling to win her confidence, at least in my own mind.

We muddled through the year and I found her to be pleasant but cautious. I found myself on the same committee with her for a great foundation in town. I had joined the committee to learn how to take my skills from my work in the diabetes community to a new level. In turn, she had learned a bit about me over that time frame and I think she trusted me.

When Jesse died, I found I was able to appreciate people in more meaningful ways. I recognized depths in people that I had never seen before. It was especially true of my feelings for this woman. Strong women are strong for a reason. Usually it's because they have climbed out of a deep hole or survived something difficult. Like all of those people walking around Target oblivious to me, she wasn't exactly wearing this inner pain on her sleeve. In time, however, she became a true friend. She told me about the death of her mother – how her own father had killed her before turning the gun on himself. It left her in sorrow at the young age of 21, alone to raise her five younger siblings. It was like that sunburn resurfacing, reminding me that loss was everywhere.

I left my meeting with this new friend. I felt very comfortable with her and had learned to separate my business self and my personal self. We laughed and joked in the midst of heated but productive business conversations and yet she could say to me, "Really, Michelle, how ARE you doing?"

I gave her a solid hug as I left that meeting – something I may not have done before Jesse's death. We had bonded through our losses.

I drove home thinking about the day. As I finished the final stretch of my drive home in bumper-to-bumper traffic, I heard a noise that made the hair on the back of my neck stand up. It was the sound of an ambulance trying to cut through impossible traffic. Not only did I look up, I started to sweat, started to panic, started to feel horrible. To me, the sight and sound of that ambulance still triggered memories of the day Jesse was clinging to life as he was driven to the hospital. The first responders were no doubt hoping they could go home that night and tell their children they had saved the life of a 13-year-old boy. Instead, all I could envision in that ambulance was a life lost.

Six months after Jesse's death, I felt that I had made strides that I could be proud of, whatever that was worth. Still, I wondered at times how I was able to stand up or stomach having a friend tell me that her daughter died suddenly or bear hearing about another friend's husband who had a heart attack. It took my breath away each time I heard stories like these, but I also felt solace in being able to help others. I felt proud by making baby steps, like being able to focus at work without having 12 meltdowns every day. Or making sure my kids were happy, that they had lunch money for the day. Or that Jesse's dad wasn't wallowing in fear and suffering. It was one day at a time, one step at a time.

When I wrote this I was sitting in the E.R. waiting for my partner to see a doctor regarding his asthma. It was the same waiting room where it all began. It was in this waiting room that my son had been diagnosed with diabetes 10 years earlier.

At the time, I thought that moment was the most traumatic, life-altering occurrence a parent could ever experience. It would change me forever, sadden me and yet make me stronger and help me find purpose in this life. Boy, was I wrong. 10 years later I went through an event that was a hundred times worse. It made Jesse's diagnosis pale in comparison.

Six months after Jesse's death, I felt that I had made strides that I could be proud of, whatever that was worth.

Still, through that experience I hoped to find the same strength and the same purpose that I recalled hoping for the first time I was in that E.R.

I know I'm not alone; there are many people that have faced losses like mine. It happens every day. Day in and day out. We question God. We question autopsies. We question Tuesdays, if that makes sense. We question a lot of things but we still exist whether we like it or not. We find joy in small things and immense sadness in others. We re-examine our lives, the way we live them and who is important to us.

That day an ambulance was not just an ambulance. I'm pretty sure that anybody who has lost a child will have their own metaphorical ambulances. All we can do is hope to survive, move forward and find joy and love in those around us. Someday, hopefully, an ambulance will just be an ambulance.

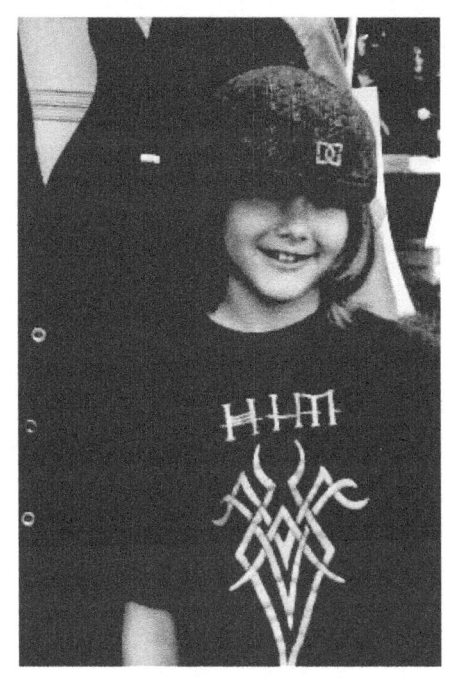

Jesse, age 12

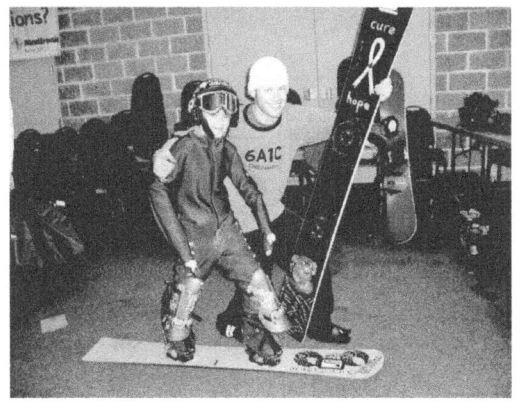

Jesse, age 8, first Riding on Insulin
camp in 2004 with Sean Busby

10
The Holidays – Anything But Merry
(10 Months, 14 days after Jesse's death)

> *"They say time heals all wounds,*
> *but that presumes*
> *the source of the grief is finite."*
> -Cassandra Clare

I HAD MADE THE DECISION WHEN I STARTED writing this book that my main purpose would be to tell about the first six months of my grieving process in the hopes that it would be of help to other people. I wrote this 10 months after Jesse died. 10 months and 14 days, to be exact, but who's counting? Oh yeah, all of us are still counting.

After Jesse died, I wondered how I would ever get through another big milestone on the calendar. The first big holiday was Valentine's Day, but that date was so close to his death that it went by without any of us even noticing. The next big day was the Super Bowl – not a holiday per se, but definitely a milestone date for Jesse. He was an avid Packers fan who would relentlessly taunt me and any other Vikings fans who would listen. Jesse would have wanted the New Orleans Saints to win that year, so we could not help but cheer the Saints on to victory while missing Jesse just that much more because he wasn't there to giggle and taunt us.

Two months later our family gathered together for Easter. I did my best to make it okay for the other kids, but I found myself immersed in a deep, dark sadness.

Before too long, it was summertime again, another time of year with lots of memories of swimming in our backyard pool. All of Jesse's friends would come over and complain about how freezing cold the water was.

We moved into fall and celebrated what would have been his 14th birthday. We chose to spend Jesse's birthday doing what we normally would have done – hanging out with his closest friends and family members, laughing and celebrating what a special person he is. Not was. Is. Somehow, his birthday remains a fond memory, not as sad as the other milestones. As I wrote this, I couldn't explain why.

Halloween and Thanksgiving came, like baby steps easing us through all the holiday milestones on the calendar. It seemed for a while like my pain was easing and I thought,

"Maybe, just maybe, I can get through all these holidays with a breath or two more."

As soon as the Thanksgiving holiday faded away, my heart grew heavier. I found myself having the same awful thoughts that I had felt during the first two months after Jesse died. I was crying all the time and couldn't seem to find joy in anything. I had thoughts of guilt and anger as to how it could be that Jesse would leave us, leave me.

As Christmas approached, I was walking through a store doing some shopping when I found myself in the ornament aisle. What started out as an okay day immediately turned to a day of intense sadness and pain. I looked at the ornaments and my only thought was, "My God, Jesse won't be here to decorate the tree. Should I still buy him an ornament? Should I still hang his Christmas stocking?"

Memories of Christmas celebrations from years past flooded my mind. I loved taking pictures of the kids standing by our Christmas tree. I loved how we set up the world's dumbest little train track around the tree skirt. I ran out of the store as quickly as I could, trying not to look like a lunatic.

During that time, I started noticing again how Jesse's death had affected me and how it was affecting my other kids. I couldn't focus at work, and I started noticing that my 10-year-old would break down and cry at school. Come to find out, he had been reading a book called *Tuck Everlasting*. There was a character in the book named Jesse and the book was about life and the afterlife. No wonder he was getting so upset. Like me, he was dealing with his own personal pain through the holiday seasons.

Jesse's friends also started reaching out to me more. They were missing him during that time of year and grieving publicly on social media.

It was at this time that I corresponded with Charlie and Mel, parents from New Zealand who had lost their 13-year-old daughter to type 1 diabetes. She had been diagnosed with the disease about the same time as Jesse. Charlie told me that he found himself going over all the phone calls he made to tell family and friends what had happened. He didn't quite understand why he obsessed over those details, but he told me it helped him deal with the approaching holidays. He needed to feel a sense of normalcy as he and his wife tried to carry on.

Right before Christmas, in the midst of our renewed feelings of pain and loss, we celebrated by completing a 100-mile bike ride through Death Valley, California. Part of that ride became a tribute to Jesse and Trent, both lost to this disease at such young ages. Trent's parents had joined me in Death Valley along with 300 other riders.

The ride program of JDRF had always been special to me. The night before the ride, the JDRF staff surprised me by speaking lovingly of Jesse and telling me that, going forward, mile 23 would be a mile ridden in silence to commemorate the date of his death. (2/3). I said, "It's for more than just Jesse. It's for everyone here who has lost someone to type 1 diabetes."

Over the years, all the riders that joined us for this event would ride that mile in silence out of respect for those who had been lost to this disease.

During any big event like this that celebrated my son's life, I found myself grieving intensely again. I wondered, "What will I do next? I have to keep busy to keep sane."

Months later, we gathered to watch a video of the weekend we spent in Death Valley. Each year we did this in celebration of all we accomplished. As much as I wanted to go to the party, I was not in the mood for it. I knew more than anything that I would be emotional and knew my friends would no doubt include a moving tribute to Jesse.

In the end, I went to the party. As I expected, whoever had created the video had included a great tribute to Jesse. I was overtaken by emotion and just wanted to escape the room. I didn't want all my grief to flow into their lives. I was sad that they couldn't just have their fun like always, that my grief had become their grief, my loss had become their loss.

I went home and later that evening I watched the video over and over, crying into the middle of the night. I couldn't help it. Selfishly, I needed to grieve over my loss. My loss.

Weeks later I received an email from a wonderful friend who had worked so hard to create the slideshow. The tribute had been backed by a Dixie Chicks tune called *Godspeed Little Man*. He kindly mentioned in his email that he wasn't sure if I had liked the video because I hadn't reacted or said anything after watching it. It was at that moment that I figured out what was going on. In my effort to explain my reaction to his video tribute, I learned more about my own struggle. It was this: the most rewarding and thoughtful efforts – phone calls, gifts, a slideshow – were the 'rewards' that came with the most excruciating and heart-wrenching pain I could possibly feel.

As difficult as it was at times to accept these gifts, they were appreciated. They were worth receiving. I wanted the givers to know and understand that the receivers might be so overcome with emotion that a response or thanks might go unsaid at the time.

My friends from New Zealand felt much the same way. Charlie told me on one occasion that somebody had left a calendar in their mailbox that their daughter had started but had not finished. At the time, he put it aside because it was too painful to look at, but he knew that at some point he would hang it up somewhere.

All those gifts we received meant everything to us. They would remain small memories that we could cling to over the years.

I kept thinking, "What the hell is wrong with me?" I thought I had been doing better, but I was feeling like I had months ago. I understood that the ebb and flow of grief and emotion would continue for a long time. I knew that seeing a boy in a store that looked like Jesse could trigger a three-hour crying jag. That getting a holiday card from a well-meaning family would conjure up thoughts of, "I'll never take a family picture again because my family is no longer whole." I knew it would pass; I knew Christmas wouldn't last all year, thank God.

We pulled up at mile 23 and stopped. Our local team gathered together, took some pictures and remembered our boys. It was very hard to do, but it felt so good to be with people who loved us, cared about our boys and were invested in our cause to help find a cure.

So, how did I handle Christmas? I realized Christmas was the most difficult holiday to handle because it was that time of year when everyone gathered together no matter what. And I realized it was also the last time our family had all been together and had a damn good time.

In the end, we decorated our tree with the kids and laughed and followed all our normal traditions. We hung

Jesse's stocking like we always did and always will. We still wondered who the hell had taken a bite out of the ornament that looked like a cookie. We finally pinned the blame on Jesse because he wasn't there to defend himself. We ended with a screeching rendition of *Grandma Got Run Over by a Reindeer* on the CD player in honor of Jesse's presence. It's all we could do, remember him, remember the good times with smiles and giggles all around. Then it was on to the next milestone holiday.

MICHELLE BAUER

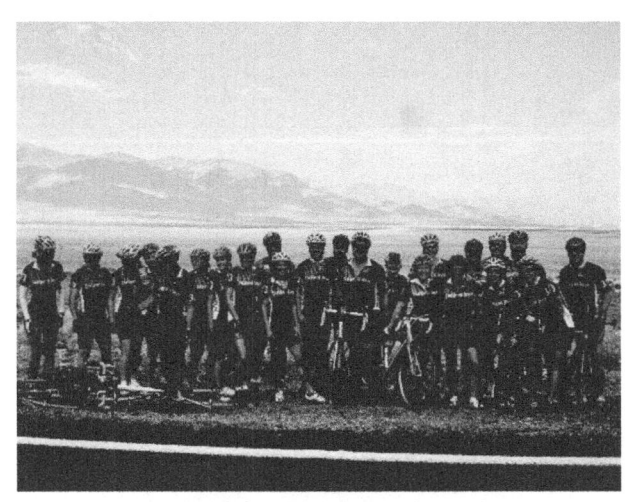

2010, Death Valley, CA, the first Mile 23 ridden in silence for Jesse

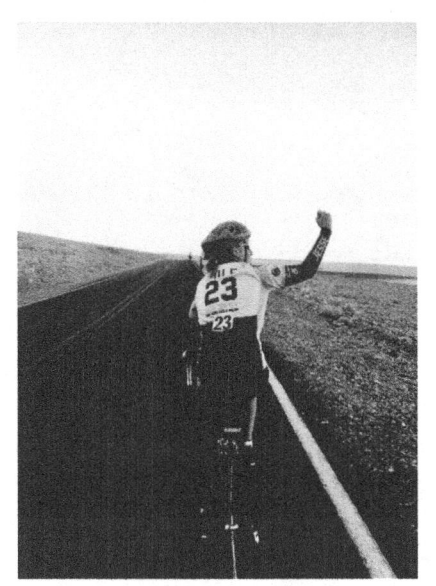

2012, Michelle returning to Death Valley with Mile 23 jersey

11
Intimacy, Relationships, Beginnings, Endings
(Five Years After Jesse's death)

"Have enough courage to trust love one more time and always one more time."
-Maya Angelou

IT TOOK SEVERAL YEARS TO BEGIN WRITING this chapter. I guess I was busy living life and finding my way. It was easier to reflect on my past relationships when some time had passed. I had time to look back and better comprehend what I had allowed to happen.

After Jesse died, I read a short book on grief. The basic message that I took away from that book was simple: "Don't make changes in your current relationship for at least a year as you may not be thinking and seeing clearly." I was in a bad relationship when Jesse died. We had been living together for about nine months and I was bound and determined to make the relationship work. After all, I had failed at my marriage with Jesse's dad. I felt as if I owed it to myself, my partner and my kids to make this one work. It became clear that the relationship was not a healthy one, and I had started to confide in my friends that I wanted out. On the day Jesse died, I did not find myself leaning on him for any kind of support. Actually, as the years passed, some of my friends told me that on that dreaded day he had pointed his finger at me and blamed me for his death. To this day, my friends have never told me exactly what he said or did. I told them not to tell me as I didn't think I could handle the pain of knowing what he said.

I remember waking up the day after Jesse died, feeling empty. He tried to support me that morning, but during the days that followed he became more and more distant. He would make jealous comments about old boyfriends who had contacted me to lend support. He would tell me I was paying too much attention to this person or that person. Looking back I can't help but think, "My God! What was wrong with him?" On the day of the funeral I wasn't sure what his role should be. Should he stand by my side? It didn't feel right, but I had him stand next to me as we greeted people. I don't know if it was the right thing to do, but that was the choice I made at the time.

Four days after the funeral I was hit with a harsh reality. The days after the funeral were difficult. Everyone had gone home, and I felt totally alone. I felt sorry for myself and cried all the time. As I was sitting at the dining room table, my significant other approached me and started questioning me about some text messages I had received from an ex-boyfriend. In one text the friend had said, "I love you," and "I wish I was there."

I had responded, "I love you, and I wish you were here too." It was an innocent expression of friendship – nothing more. I had received hundreds of texts from other people with the same message. I needed that kind of support to help me get through the pain. Yet my significant other interpreted this as though I wanted to be with this other man. I was so exhausted and full of pain that all I was capable of doing at the time was protect my other children. I told him that my children had been through enough and I did not want him to cause them any more pain. Why couldn't this man see my pain? Why couldn't he support me in ways that I needed? The painful answer was that he was incapable of helping me, but it would

Out of loss can come friendship and love.

take another full year before I was able to find the strength to leave.

Over the next year, our relationship remained tumultuous. There was constant arguing and finger pointing. I was cold. I was numb. I just didn't care. I was living one day at a time trying to put one foot in front of the other. He continued his threatening behavior until finally I picked up the phone and arranged for a new place for my kids and me to live. My family and friends, once again, were a tremendous support. I don't know what I would have done without them.

That decision did not come easily. In fact, I went to counseling beforehand. After a number of sessions with a wonderful therapist, including one with my significant other, my counselor told me that this man was incapable of owning his own issues. She said that she felt I was handling my personal grief and pain and owning my faults in the relationship. It was at this point that I gave myself permission to leave.

Over the next year, I settled into my new home with my children. It was a year of healing and a year of learning to handle pain on my own. What I discovered was that I had spent so much time grieving the loss of my son and the loss of a healthy relationship that it was freeing to finally be able to just grieve the loss of my son. I finally found peace after leaving that unhealthy relationship. During that year I was also able to focus more on my other kids and have fun with them in the simple things. Sure, I sometimes struggled with the fact that there were fewer plates at the dinner table, but the quality of the food was better.

I did go on a handful of dates and attempted some new relationships, but nothing felt right. I realized I wasn't much different from any other woman in her 40s looking for a decent guy to spend time with. I wasn't that special.

Throughout this time, I would still have wonderful conversations with Jesse's dad about dating, love and where we would go from here. Jesse's dad said it perfectly when he told me he had only been dating casually because his heart, like mine, was still broken.

He didn't see how he could possibly share his life with somebody who had not met Jesse, who didn't understand the pain of losing a child. We were on the same page as we entered the unknown.

During this awkward dating process I went to my 25th high school class reunion. I had decided to throw on a dress and go see some old friends. I arrived at the venue, looked around and saw many familiar faces – faces that did not even know I had a son, let alone a son that had died. I took a deep breath, ordered a glass of wine and waded into the crowd.

I was chatting with a friend who had sat next to me in biology class. I looked up and saw a man I had dated during my senior year of high school and smiled at him. I had not seen him once in 25 years. I'll admit there were times over the years when I thought, "I wonder whatever happened to…" We pointed at each other and I remember saying, "Hey, I know you." We chatted briefly and asked about each other's families and decided we would sit together at dinner.

As we sat down to eat, I remember a couple of things. First of all, I noticed that this guy, who used to be loud and outgoing, was now quiet and thoughtful. It was like our roles from high school had been reversed over the past 25 years. Naturally, at some point he asked the question I had been dreading. "So, how many kids do you have?"

I gathered strength and spilled the lines I had rehearsed and spoken so many times before. I'll never forget the look on his face. It was full of compassion and even a hint of pain. He told me he didn't realize how prevalent diabetes was.

In a bitter stroke of irony, as soon as he said that, two other people at the table took out their blood glucose monitors and tossed them on the table. Our own classmates had been affected by the same disease that took my son.

During the rest of the evening we crossed paths here and there. He told me about the painful end to his marriage, and I immediately found myself attracted to his honesty.

The conversations we had that night really helped me. Some of the pain was lifted from my heart. I didn't even realize it until I started writing about it. Our connection that night was short and it never became permanent, but I realized that I was deserving of kindness and friendship and joy. Looking back on that night, I still find it funny that I shared grief and happiness with somebody who didn't even know my child.

I wrote this on an airplane flying at 30,000 feet. Two songs that I love played in the background. Both always reminded me of Jesse: *Don't Stop Believin'* by Journey and *You and Me* by the Dave Matthews Band. Jesse was still part of me and I felt as if he approved of what I was doing. It was time to tell the rest of the story.

JESSE WAS HERE

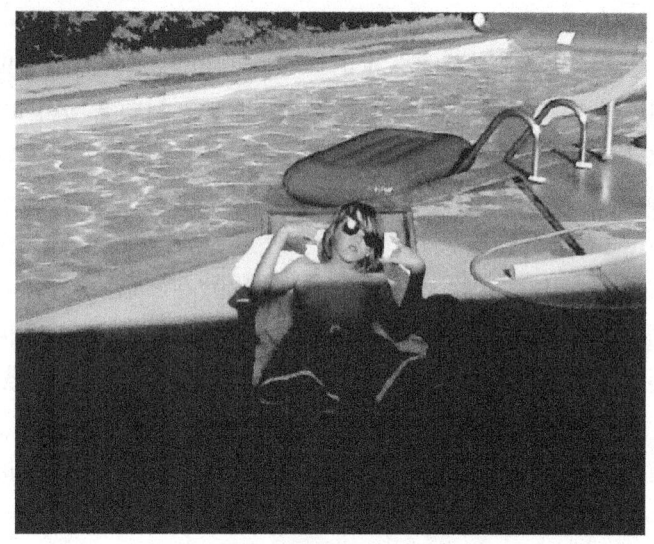

Jesse, age 13, chillin' by the pool

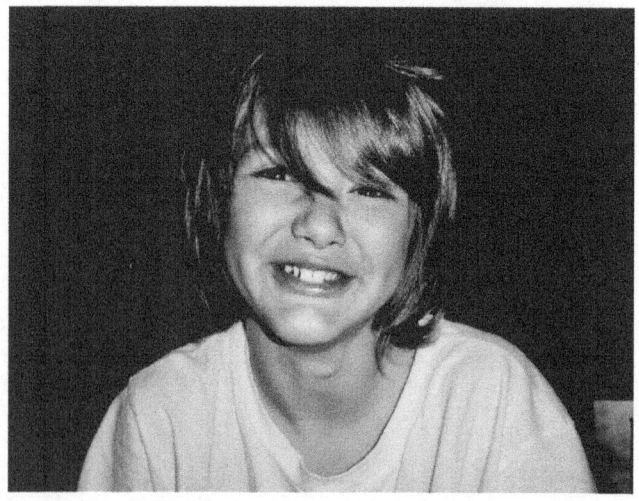

Jesse, age 13, best smile on the planet

12
The Worst Day of My Life
(Six months after Jesse's death)

> *"Today is not your worst day, that day is over."*
> *-Sara Rankin*

BY NOW, MOST OF YOU ARE PROBABLY WONdering, "So, what actually happened?"

The day Jesse died was the day my life changed forever. I'd like to tell you that I was brave enough to write this as it happened or shortly thereafter. However, I was in shock, numb, unable to even look at the form sitting on the kitchen table that I was supposed to fill out, let alone write about my thoughts.

No, I wrote this chapter six months after the day it all happened. I didn't have the courage to write it until then.

There was so much pain and sadness. I couldn't dwell on it; I couldn't even *think* about that day for months. Even as I wrote this, I struggled to put my words in order and write them down. Still, I hope that now these words will help – help others understand what happened, help others heal. I wasn't sure I'd ever get to a better place or that I'd be able to go for a bike ride or go to work or enjoy a glass of wine with a friend.

For anybody else that has gone through this, I'm sure these feelings are shared. I'd like to tell you that you will get to a better place. You will be able to go for a bike ride, go to work or enjoy a glass of wine with a friend. Even if we never meet, we will always be connected as we try to make sense of the losses we suffered.

I'm not sure why I waited until this point in my story to explain what happened the day Jesse died. I know people are curious, and that's okay. Honestly, it's cathartic for me to tell the story again.

Jesse was diagnosed with type 1 diabetes at the age of three. He mostly lived his life as a normal kid. He was well-liked and respected by just about everybody. Throughout the time that he had the disease, he was always an advocate for others and wanted to help find a cure.

On February 2, 2010, we were sitting around the dinner table as usual. For dinner that night we had homemade chicken soup and steak over potatoes, a meal that Jesse always loved. I have not recreated that meal once since he died; I didn't think I could enjoy it. There was some banter at the table, and my kids were teasing me about my upcoming bike ride in Lake Tahoe. I had been doing sponsored rides in Jesse's honor for nearly 10 years in an effort to raise money for the Juvenile Diabetes Research Foundation. Jesse, like he often did, flipped his hair back, rolled his eyes and said, "Sheesh, mom, seriously, get a grip! We know you do stuff in the diabetes world for me."

After we finished dinner, Jesse and I settled in to watch Kindergarten Cop with his younger brother. We spent the evening together, laughing. Since our nights hanging out together as a family were rare, I let them stay up late even though there was school in the morning.

At 6:30 the next morning I woke Jesse up like I did every school morning. He said, "I don't feel very good today, mom." After 10 years of dealing with his disease, I knew this was just another bad diabetes morning, but that it was nothing to worry about. Like any person with type 1 diabetes, he had days when his blood sugars got out of whack and that never felt good. I said, "How are your blood sugars?"

He said, "Fine."

Thinking that he might just be overtired and didn't want to go to school, I was a little irritated. I said, "I can't stay home with you all day. I have a meeting to go to an hour away, so you can call me if you need me."

I got ready like any other normal day. I worked from home quite often, but on this particular day I had an important meeting with a client that I just couldn't miss.

I went to the meeting and found myself talking proudly about Jesse as they told me about some new initiatives in the diabetes world. The meeting went well, and afterwards, my coworker and I got in our car and left.

I was picking up a new car on the way home. My colleague dropped me off at the bank to pick it up and, while waiting in line, I thought to text Jesse's dad to let him know that he had stayed home from school. I asked if he could pick him up at my house rather than have him take the bus directly from school to his house. I got that okayed and then called my boyfriend to tell him the new car was driving nicely and that I should be home soon.

A little while later, Jesse's dad called me back and informed me that when he sent Jesse's little brother into the house to get him, the house was empty. He had checked his room and the couch and he wasn't there. His dad didn't think it was all that strange since we lived less than a mile apart. He thought that maybe Jesse had walked over to his place at some point.

It was at that very moment that I knew something was wrong. Call it a mother's intuition, but a feeling of dread and panic shot through my entire body. I just knew something was very wrong. I asked Jesse's dad to immediately drive back to my house. Instead of turning around, he chose to check his house first. I can never blame him for doing that. He is a good man and who could have known the unthinkable might be happening?

As he drove back to my house to check again for Jesse, I called my boyfriend and told him something was wrong. Very wrong. Then I started calling some of my close friends. I have to be honest, it's very hard for me to accurately remember exactly what happened. I can't remember who I called first or what time it was. I was panicking and thinking to myself, "What if? What if?"

I tried calling his dad again. No answer. No answer. No answer. No answer. I knew he must be talking to somebody else because I kept getting sent directly to his voicemail.

Sheer panic. I kept calling. No answer. No answer. And then the worst answer. Finally his dad picked up and started screaming that Jesses wasn't breathing and that the EMTs were at my house working on him.

I can't remember all the details of what happened next. I'm not sure I want to. But I do remember screaming the whole way back to my house, begging for his dad to save him. Begging him to tell the EMTs to not let him die! I just kept saying, "NO! NO! NO!"

I remember the battery on my phone going low and I didn't want to hang up. I was terrified. I called my friends. I called my boyfriend screaming, "Jesse is dead!" Even before I got there, I just knew the worst had happened. I was still 40 minutes from home, counting the miles and the minutes, knowing that every second was critical. I started trying to mentally prepare myself for the worst. I just knew he was gone.

I finally arrived at home. I drove up the cul-de-sac, not wanting to get out of my car. I didn't want to face the EMTs, the detectives or my friends. I finally walked into the house and saw both familiar and unfamiliar faces. I collapsed to the ground. It was dreadful. My phone rang again and it was Jesse's dad. He was following the ambulance on its way the hospital. "He's got a pulse," he said. I felt nothing.

A female detective named Kris was there next to me. She said, "That's good, Michelle."

I screamed back at her, "What do you know? I'm not stupid! He's dead!" Little did I know that the people in the room had already been told to be prepared for the worst. The room was devoid of hope.

I was driven to the hospital. I was numb. I can't even describe the feeling.

I know a million calls had been made by family and friends, so by the time I got to the hospital the place was full of familiar faces. I ran to the emergency room where I was finally reunited with Jesse. There were tubes everywhere and a lot of grim looking faces. Looking back, I know I was in a state of shock. I looked at my two other children and couldn't bring myself to be honest with them, to tell them that their brother was dying.

The doctors took us aside and told us that his body had been through too much. They were preparing us for the worst. They transferred him upstairs where family and friends could gather to say their goodbyes. I look back now and remember how everyone assumed their own roles. Friends called other friends to break the news, my sister fell apart, Jesse's sister was strong and ready to help everyone deal with this loss, finding love and goodness in the moment of his death. I took the role of decision maker. So strange, all of it. I had to walk out of the room several times. I was in a state of disbelief and felt like I couldn't breathe, hoping that I would walk back into the room and hear someone say, "He opened his eyes! He's going to be okay!" It never happened.

True to Jesse's character, he was thoughtful in his death just like he was thoughtful in his life. He didn't cling to life. It was if he wanted to save us from that pain. He gave us just enough time to say good-bye before he let go and slipped away peacefully.

As I stood there holding his little hand, not wanting to let him go, the coroner came in and started bombarding us with questions. It was invasive and insulting. "How could we leave a 13-year-old boy home alone? Was there any insulin in the house?" Ridiculous questions from a man who didn't understand diabetes and certainly didn't know Jesse. To this day, I still hate that man for what he did. I have similar feelings for the nurse who had been pushing fluids into my dying son. When a new nurse came into the room she asked the nurse attending to Jesse, "How's your day going?"

"Pretty good, so far," the nurse answered.

Then I heard somebody say the word 'autopsy.' The word seemed to crawl up out of the coroner's mouth. He told us it needed to be done, that we had no choice. The thought of my son being physically ripped apart was excruciating. He was my baby. I couldn't bear the thought of Jesse in a cold room being torn apart, only to have them find nothing conclusive.

I was numb when we left the hospital. As we were driving home, we realized we needed to get gas. It was so strange that we still had to do normal things like that in what had just become a very un-normal world. There I stood pumping gas with these words on my lips, "My son just died."

I started sobbing. My son had just died. I had nothing left. When I got home, I walked into the house and climbed into bed. I had let the other kids go home with their dad as I knew he would need them. I curled up under the covers and cried myself to sleep.

When I woke up the next morning, my first thought was, "My son is dead," and I started crying again. I finally got up and saw Jesse's ski trip form lying on the kitchen table. I grabbed it and held on to it like it was a piece of gold. It was a part of him. I walked through the house, numb, and was grateful when I heard the doorbell ring.

The first of many friends had arrived. There stood Amy, ready to help me deal with the first day after losing my son. That day remains a blur in my memory. People were coming and going, bringing food, crying with me. I was not only exhausted by my own grief, I was exhausted by theirs. They were grieving with me and for me. I remember wanting to climb back into bed, curl up and cry, but I also remember being grateful that there were other people around. From the very beginning, I knew I couldn't wallow in lonesome grief. I had to cry; I had to talk; I had to let it out.

When my extended family arrived, I told them I was worried about Jesse's dad. His extended family had yet to arrive to support him. My mother finally went to his house to pick him up and bring him and the kids back to my house to grieve together. He didn't want to set foot in that house again. After all, it would always be the place where his son died. I couldn't blame him, yet he knew it was good for all of us to be together.

On Thursday, just a couple days after Jesse died, Amy told me that we needed to pick a funeral home. A funeral home?

What the hell did I know about funeral homes? Together, we picked one out and we set up a planning appointment for the next day. I felt relieved not to have to deal with that by myself. My friends and family stayed close by, made dinner for me and then I drank myself to sleep.

That night I had a horrible dream about Jesse. In my dream he was lying on a couch wearing his favorite blue hoodie, covered by a blanket. His eyes were slits. They looked like the same cold, empty eyes from the day he died. He kept telling me that he was so cold. I was grateful to see him alive but awoke to the reality of his death once again. My brain was playing a cold trick on me, allowing me to see him and touch him in my mind's eye. I hated myself for having that dream. Those images still tortured me six months later, but I'm grateful that dreams like that didn't reappear after that night.

Friday morning we woke up to go to the funeral home to make final plans. Behind the scenes, friends had already started a memorial fund for us. I already had some ideas in my head on how best to respect everyone's wishes. I brought Sandy and Amy, two of my best friends, along for support, knowing that it would be difficult to be objective.

Jesse's dad had been adamant about the fact that he wanted a private funeral. I was adamant that we were going to need the biggest church in town. I also wanted a church near Jesse's school which would allow less fortunate kids to walk over directly from school. There would be people coming who had never met Jesse, flying in from as far away as London because he had inspired them over the years. This was just one of the decisions that had to be made.

My 16-year-old daughter had been loud and vocal saying that Jesse wouldn't want an open casket. My mother said people would expect a viewing so they could say goodbye. There I stood with my own beliefs being forced to think about how to make everyone happy. It wasn't easy.

We sat together planning the funeral. We handed over our son's clothes with tears in our eyes. I watched Jesse's dad as he observed the support my friends gave me. They made sure we did not have to cut a check to pay for the arrangements that day. They were taking care of everything out of love for me and respect for Jesse. As Jesse's dad saw all this love and support, I could feel him soften. He was moved by how everybody worked together to spare us. We decided to have an open casket for family and friends who didn't get to say goodbye at the hospital. Afterward, we would close the casket for the wake and the funeral and cremate Jesse's remains after it was all said and done.

We chose Monday for the funeral. We would have to get through the weekend, and I remember feeling relieved at the delay. I knew that day would loom heavy, however.

We spent Friday evening at Jesse's dad's house supporting him and spending time with family and friends. It was a night where we shared memories, tears and laughter. Jesse's death had brought so many people back together that normally would never have found a reason to talk to each other. Jesse's dad took me aside later in the evening. He wanted to make sure that we would support each other moving forward. We promised that we would never blame each other or ourselves. I was grateful for that moment.

The weekend passed quickly. I received a card in the mail from a friend named Sarah whose 23-year-old son Austin had died two years before in a car accident while suffering from high blood sugars. Her words were so wise, that I find it important to share them. She stated, "Today is not your worst day; your worst day is over." I cried, yet I knew she was right. I also knew that until the funeral was over, day one after the worst day could not truly begin. Then, and only then, could the healing begin.

Monday, the day of the funeral, had arrived.

I woke up feeling sick to my stomach. The horrible day was here. I was going to have to face the public and let my grief show to the world whether I was ready or not. I put on my dress after getting the kids ready. It was time to drive two blocks to the church. I leaned over to my partner with tears in my eyes in my new car, the car that I now loathed, the car that had become a symbol of my son's death, and said, "I'm not ready. I don't want to do this. Don't make me go." I was so scared.

The casket was looming when we entered the church. I had always been the type of person who believed the body was the garage to the soul. I never believed the body to be anything to look at during a funeral since the soul was no longer there, so why stare?

If it hadn't been my son, I would not have looked at the body that lay before me. Yet, I felt this horrible gnawing in my body about what people would think. How could I not go say good-bye to my own son? What a horrible mother! Yes, those thoughts went through my mind. I didn't want the last memory of my son to be him lying in a casket, lifeless.

The decision was made for me in a glorious and natural way. I had arrived at the church and saw my other kids. They were ready to go view Jesse's body, so how could I turn them away? How could I not join them? I had to be strong. I walked up to the casket holding my daughter's hand. I think I needed her strength more than she needed mine. I'll never forget the feeling that coursed through my body, because I watched my daughter experience the exact same feeling. "It isn't him," she said.

For me and my daughter, that simply was not my son. I was relieved. Yes, I was actually relieved because I believed throughout the funeral that my son's presence was there. There was no doubt about that. He was not in that coffin, not in that body. I was grateful when it was time to close the casket. In fact, as I wrote this, I squinted my eyes shut, not ever wanting to see that dreadful image again as long as I lived.

The church filled quickly with over 1,000 people offering condolences. As Jesse's dad and I stood at the front of the church, we realized it was going to be the longest day of our lives. As each person greeted us, there was new grief, new suffering, new loss, both ours and theirs. Instead of only feeling the support of others, I believe we also offered support to them. It was a strange feeling.

I watched as a church full of 13-year-old children leaned on each other and wept openly. I knew their lives were forever changed. I also knew the people in that church would be forever changed as they witnessed 13-year-old pallbearers escort their best friend out the door. That's a sight I hope to never see again in this lifetime. I was filled with pride for my son and for all the friends whose lives he had touched. There was so much love.

Jesse's sister and one of his best friends wrote beautiful eulogies for the funeral:

"My name is Sean, and Jesse was my friend. He was everyone's friend. He was everyone's little

brother. He was mine too. We did things that brothers do. I taught him how to snowboard. We talked, we emailed, I heard about his guitar lessons. We shared like brothers do. We shared having diabetes together.

I was diagnosed with my diabetes during Children's Congress 2003, an event that ultimately saved my life when I had lost all hope. For those that may not know, Jesse was part of this Children's Congress and was one of the kids that helped me not to give up. Jesse came into my life to turn it around and help me live with my diabetes. He came to me to make an impact and he was and always will be my guardian angel.

From that Children's Congress, Jesse's story and others' stories helped me turn my life around and dedicate it to helping children and teens with type 1 diabetes through my snowboarding career. On my path to bettering myself and to give back to kids who inspired me to keep competing and snowboarding, I met a strong-willed mother named Michelle. She had organized a foundation to help her child, Jesse, and millions of other children who had type 1 diabetes. Michelle's foundation was there to give back to those with type 1 through sports and sport camps. Michelle and I quickly became best friends and her son became a major influence behind my Riding on Insulin Snowboarding Camps.

My first official Midwest Riding on Insulin Snowboarding Camp was held in Wisconsin where I got to finally meet Michelle and her amazing son Jesse. Since that day, a beautiful friendship transpired. Michelle and Jesse gave me the will and the tools to put on my snowboarding camps around the world for multiple children's hospitals and foundations that serve kids with diabetes. These camps have since been put on in New Zealand and across the entire USA. My biggest inspiration to turn these camps global and at a national level came from Michelle's son Jesse who was also my biggest fan.

Jesse was instantly hooked on snowboarding from our very first Midwest camp. He found a sense of freedom by strapping his two feet into a board that took him away from his life that was filled with insulin injections, finger pricks, insulin reactions and carb counting. I remember riding up on the chairlift and having a conversations about school and diabetes. I remember how he bombed down the hill like a maniac and the extra-large gloves that he was wearing that day and my goggles. Jesse was a funny, funny kid and was all about having a good time. On my last visit, Jesse and his friend Paul and I trash talked each other during a game of mini-sized pool. While Jesse and Paul racked all the balls away, I worked on my next excuse for why I was so horrible at the game and why a couple of young kids could put away an adult in such a game. Filled with ridiculous excuses, we had a great time that I will never forget.

Since my first Wisconsin camp, Jesse and Michelle have become family to me. We have hosted numerous other Riding on Insulin camps in Wisconsin together, and I would stay with Michelle and Jesse whenever I was in the area. Jesse has always kept me up to date on his "girlfriends," when he went snowboarding, when he broke his arm skateboarding, his scars, his guitar lessons, and of course any bad days that he was having with his diabetes. I also kept Jesse in the loop with things such as girlfriend advice, college, snowboarding, my skateboard injuries and my diabetes. Jesse and Michelle were my main diabetes support group, and Jesse was my little homie. While Jesse went on living his life with type 1, Michelle and I worked on bettering the camps and networking with many well-known foundations in order to give back to more kids just like Jesse throughout the Midwest. Looking now at the bigger picture, this is what Jesse would want, at least from me. Jesse wasn't selfish and was all about making sure kids just like him were also looked after and cared for. Jesse cared for his family, especially his little brother and his older sister. Jesse was a gift that we got to barrow until he would be sent on to do bigger things. Jesse has enabled all of us to live on in his spirit and he will now always be our co-pilot. I am sure that Jesse has a mission for all of us, and I urge all of us to find that mission so that we can live on in Jesse's spirit and memory.

We now have a new star in our sky, there to protect us and guide us. This news is absolutely devastating to all of us and I am sure when we are all with Jesse one day, he will ask us what all this fuss was about. While we are here mourning, he is probably up there skating an awesome skatepark, slashing a rad powder cloud on his snowboard, or jamming out with many rock stars. I will live my life with a new motto: 'Jesse would do it.' Whenever I have doubts about diabetes, I will think about what Jesse would do and what the bigger picture is all about.

He inspired me and saved my life when I was first diagnosed. I am since making my commitment to Jesse – that after a temporary hold on Riding on Insulin – Riding on Insulin will return to help diabetic children and teens of the Midwest and the rest of the world by this time next year. Jesse is my hero and I will miss him deeply. I love you, Jesse, and you will always be in my heart every time I strap into my board. Go ride those powdery clouds, my man. I will miss you so much. Your song has ended, but your melody lingers on."

Your biggest fan, Sean

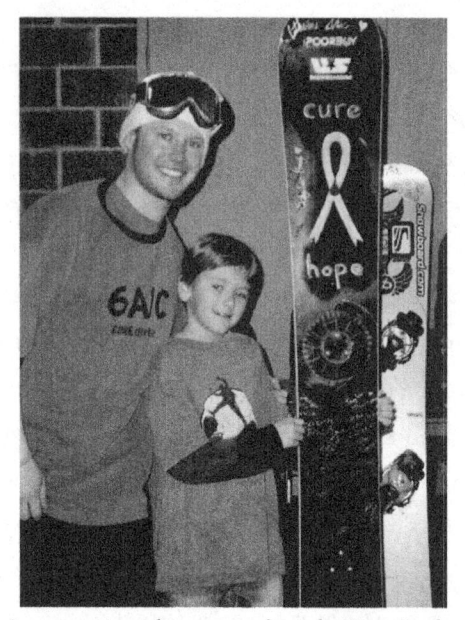

Jesse, age 8, with pro snowboarder Sean Busby

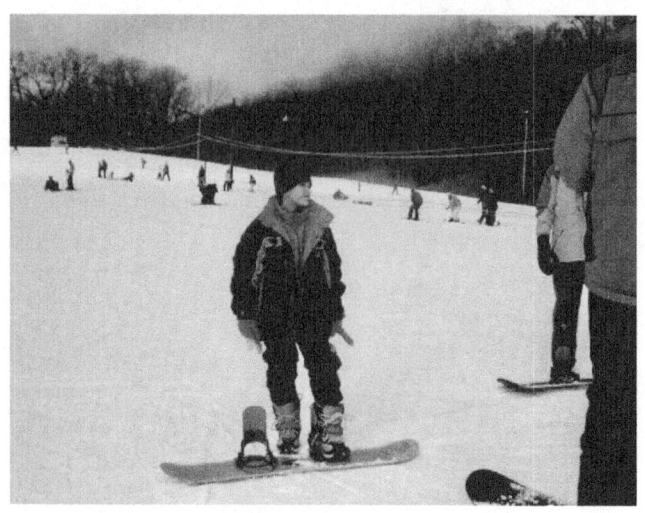

Jesse, age 8, at first Riding on Insulin camp

"Jesse was more than just my brother, he was my best friend too. We told each other just about everything that we did. He had so many great things to do down here, but I know he will do better things up there. It's really hard for me to cry about him anymore. I know that everyone will miss him SO MUCH but whenever I remember this kid, I can only smile and laugh. He jumped on any excuse to do something stupid and pointless.

Ever since Jesse was born we were extremely close, but as we got older we got even closer. I saw him every day and I'm going to miss going home and playing Family Feud and Rockband together after school. Jesse is not just my little brother. He was everyone's little brother, everyone's kid, everyone's friend. Whenever my friends came over, they didn't just come over to see me, they came for Jesse and some serious laughing that he brought us.

When he found something that made us laugh, he would not give up on that joke, even if it meant all of us on the floor, out of breath, crying from laughing so hard. I was his older sister, but a lot of the time he was my older brother. He helped me whenever I needed him. I quit ballet to join hockey with him. He pushed me to do better in school, and to do better with everything else I did. I admit that I was jealous of how amazing he was, but who wouldn't be jealous of him? He had everything.

He had the talent to do anything he really wanted to do, and he would work on one thing until he did it perfectly. He had the hair, the looks, the humor. All the ladies fell head over heels just to be with him, and I understand why. Jesse has touched everyone that met him, more people than I even thought was possible for a 13-year-old to know. And when I see everyone who came to support him and my family, I can't thank them enough or thank them the way I want to.

Jesse got diabetes when he was only three, and as soon as he got it, he wanted to pretend it wasn't there. He just wanted to live a normal little boy life. Unfortunately, we lost the battle with diabetes in this case, but I know that we have not lost the war.

We all love Jesse and he will always be with us and in our hearts."

Samantha

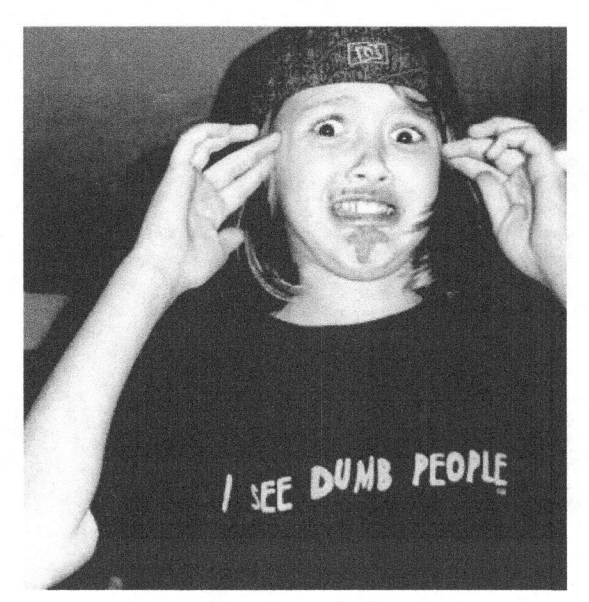

Jesse, age 13, always the funny and
handsome little brother

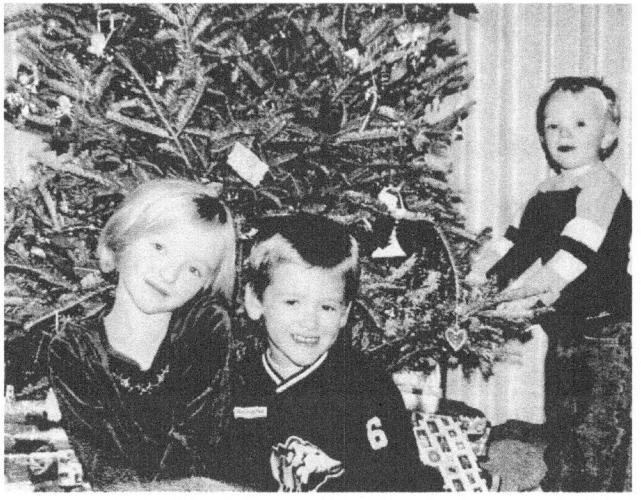

Jesse, age 6, Christmas with his siblings

JESSE WAS HERE

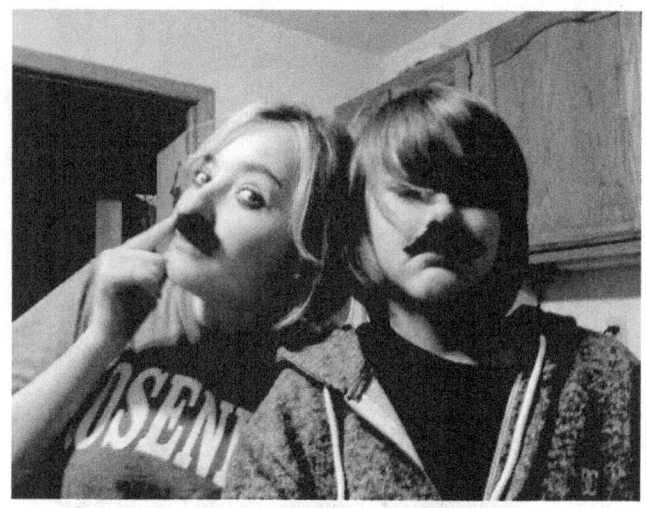

Jesse, age 13, with Sam…thick as thieves

Day 1 – The Day After the Funeral

I had a second Day 1 of the grieving process. For me, I couldn't truly start to move forward until the funeral was over. My whole life was in limbo until I shook the last hand, gave the last hug and said good-bye to an exhausting, brutal time in my life.

Day 2 – The Healing Process

I had no idea how much the words, "we need to do an autopsy" would hurt until they were said to me. I'm not sure if coroners in general are not taught good bedside manner, but the coroner that presided at Jesse's death certainly did not have it. It felt as if he descended into the room just moments after Jesse took his last breath. I refused to let go of his hand – not that anybody was trying to stop me. It was like I was fighting a battle inside my own head. "I won't let go; I'm not ready."

It felt to me like the coroner was a vulture. I was sick, I was sad and I was being asked questions like, "Why was he home alone? Did you have insulin in the house?" Then, without pausing, he said, "We need to do an autopsy whether you like it or not." When the word "autopsy" came out of his mouth, I admit, it just created another layer of pain and dread. They were going to cut up my baby, my little boy. Did they know what they were asking of me? He was perfect. Wasn't his death bad enough?

Over the next few weeks I came to hate that coroner for his crass questions and his inaccurate perception of the disease that took my son's life. I was trusting this man to tell us what went wrong, and I will always believe he really didn't know – he was incapable of such certainty.

Then I heard the words "organ donation." Oh, man, I remembered how I had acted all strong and brave at the DMV when they asked if I wanted be an organ donor. I grabbed the orange sticker and said, "Heck yeah!"

Well, let me tell you, I was unprepared for the moment when someone asked me if I wanted to donate Jesse's tissue. I had no time to really think about the answer, though I knew somebody else was waiting for a heart, a kidney, an eye. I looked at my ex-husband with a pained look, and thought about them taking my precious son's organs. I didn't want them to. I was about to say no. I saw his dad starting to say no and then I said, "Wait. We have to. We just have to. What if one of our kids needed that transplant? What if it was Jesse who was dying and we could save him with someone else's dying son's organ? We'd want it; we'd beg for it." In the end, we agreed.

> *I was filled with pride for my son and for all the friends whose lives he had touched. There was so much love.*

Then we were hit with a final slap in the face when we were told that his body had been so ravaged that they could only use his tissue, but we were okay with that. Still, it felt like somebody was stealing pieces of the boy I brought into this world. I had to think rationally, whether I liked it or not.

MICHELLE BAUER

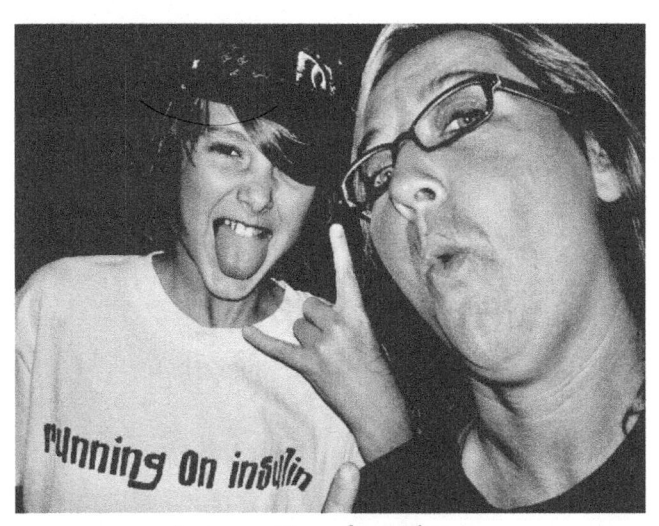

Jesse, age 13, goofing with mom

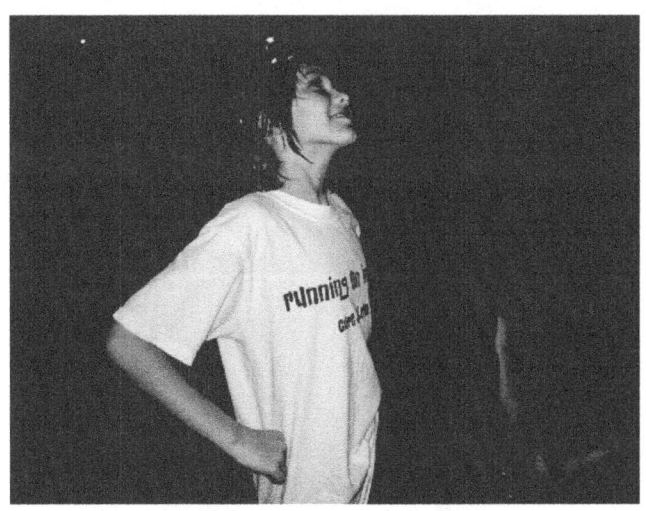

Jesse, age 13, last vacation together

13
Compartmentalized Living

(Five years after Jesse's death)

*"Life can only be understood backwards;
it must be lived forwards."*
-Soren Kierkegaard

YEARS AGO I WAS IN A TUMULTUOUS RELAtionship with a very fun man who taught me much about spontaneity and living life. I will never forget an intense conversation with him about how men and women are different and how men compartmentalized their emotions, thoughts, feelings and actions in order to function. Case in point, if he was spending a great deal of time focusing on his feelings and spending time with me, his work would suffer. On the other hand, if he would spend all of his thoughts, energy and emotion on his work, he would feel like he wasn't giving enough to our relationship.

I could never understand that thought process. Like many women, I considered myself to be a multi-tasker. I could fit all facets of my life into my head and heart and function just fine.

Five years after Jesse died, he would have been 18 years old and graduating from high school. I admit it was difficult to watch his friends write on social media about their plans for graduation, getting into colleges, even simple things like growing taller.

I watched that year as Jesse's little brother surpassed him in age and height. I also watched his sister turn 21. The kids were more a symbol of life moving on – scratch that – life moving FORWARD – than any calendar could have provided me. It was a sharp reminder that life goes on. Those thoughts put a smile on my face.

During the five years that passed after Jesse died, I gradually saw myself grieve, grow and change.

During the five years that passed after Jesse died, I gradually saw myself grieve, grow and change. Some of it was so gradual that I barely noticed it was happening and could only reflect upon it later. Relationships came and went, some good and some not so good. From each one I learned more about my own strengths and weaknesses, and I learned to allow myself joy in this new version of my life. I knew my life would never be the same. I knew it then. I know it now. Today, when people ask me where I'm at, sometimes I catch myself saying, "I have never been happier."

At first I cringed when those words came out of my mouth. How could I say that? My son is gone. My heart is not the same. I wondered how others perceived that comment. Did they wonder, "What a terrible thing to say!" Or were they thinking, "Good for her." Until then, I didn't know how to explain how I could utter those words, words that I never thought I'd be able to say.

I was staring out the window of a plane on my way to another Riding on Insulin camp in California, a camp that Jesse loved. It occurred to me – I lived a compartmentalized life. It was how I learned to cope. It was how I learned to keep living. It was how I allowed myself to feel joy again. There were times when I had to fight feelings of guilt for the happy days I had, but I felt I deserved happiness again.

I had to compartmentalize the pain I felt as I drove to the airport and heard a song that reminded me of Jesse. Then, an hour later, kiss the person who had supported and loved me no matter what. I learned to cope; I learned to heal.

I know I couldn't have become the person I was without

lots of help from the amazing people who surrounded me. I also knew that there were others out there like me who were just trying to get through the next day, just trying to breathe again.

After five years, I finally understood, with minimal guilt, that the pain would always be there, but I knew there were other compartments in my life that were full of joy and happiness and belonging.

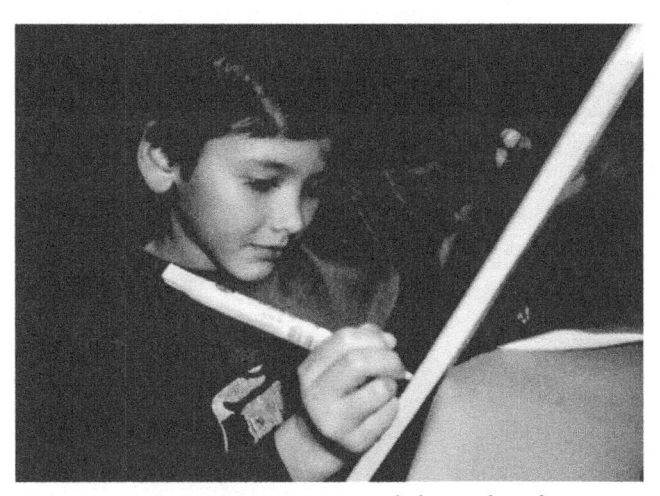

Jesse, age 8, signing Sean Busby's snowboard

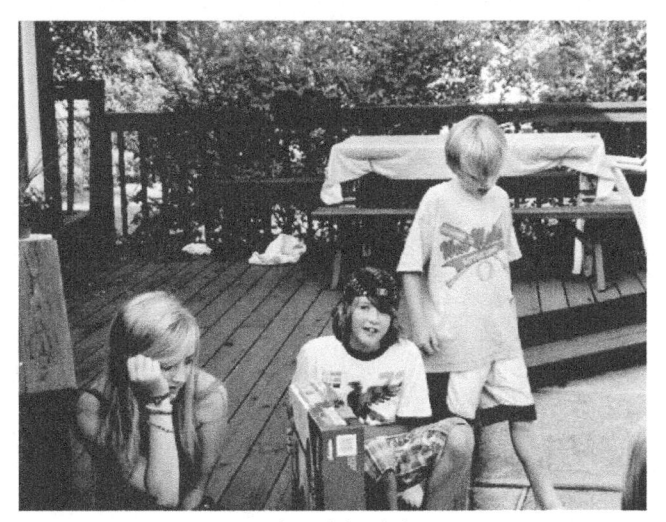

Jesse's 13th birthday

14
I Don't Care That Your Cat Died

(Written over a period of time after Jesse's death)

> *"The feeling of commiseration is the beginning of humanity."*
> *-Mencius*

FRIENDS AND FAMILY OUT THERE *ALWAYS* meant well. I knew that; I never doubted it for a second. But I had lost a child and was living through hell. There really was no method to my madness in coping with my loss. One thing I recall is that many of my closest friends kept asking, "What can we do to help?"

First of all, there was really no right thing to say. There simply wasn't. And as much as they didn't know what to say to me, I didn't know what to say to them either. It wasn't because I didn't appreciate their interest or concern, I just felt empty, sad and lost. My answer to their question should have been, "There's nothing you *can* say, really." Or, "Just saying you don't know what to say is actually saying something, so thank you." Sometimes, just being in the room with me counted for a whole lot.

If you're reading this book because someone you know has lost a loved one and you want to help, print this list of things *not* to say and give the list to everyone who may cross that person's path. These were some of the things people said to me, all well-meaning, I'm sure, but still…

"Why don't you go get a pedicure, enjoy a glass of wine and forget your troubles." I couldn't forget my troubles. I'd lost someone so dear to me that my heart literally ached. Don't get me wrong, bringing me a case of wine would have been awesome, but telling me that doing something superficial like getting a pedicure didn't make me feel better. It just didn't.

"My cat was like family. We were devastated when she died." Sorry to be harsh, but it's *not* the same. Losing a cat can't begin to compare to losing a child. The moment that starts to come out of your mouth, stop yourself.

"I lost my grandmother recently." I know you were close to your grandmother. We all are close to our grandmothers. But comparing your grandmother's death at 82 to my son's death at 13? Well, you get the idea. A full life vs. an interrupted life? No comparison, folks.

"Do you want me to take pictures at the funeral?" A resounding, "No thank you." It's not your place. Also, In case you're wondering, posting photos on social media of a funeral is indecent and thoughtless. Yes, it happened.

"He is in a better place." There were times when I was ready to hear this, but don't be offended if this is the response: "Really? Because I think this place is pretty damn great, and I wish him back, thank you very much."

"Time will heal everything." I believed this to be true, but I wasn't ready to hear it at first. As my friend Bryan said after losing his wife, "I'm tired of hearing that time will heal everything because as far as I can see, time has made the loss worse." NOTE: If you are someone who has lost a child, etc., you *are* in a place to say things like "time will heal" because you speak from experience. I found that hearing from those who had made it through a few years of grieving could confirm my feelings and give me hope that someday the pain would go away.

> *If you're reading this book because someone you know has lost a loved one and you want to help, print this list of things not to say and give the list to everyone who may cross that person's path.*

"You never really thanked me for all I did for you." Yes, a lot of people did a lot of wonderful things for me, and I appreciated them with all my heart. However, as hard as it may have been for you to not get a "thank you," you have to realize that the pain I felt was excruciating. I went to work with a smile on my face, and I pretended as if I was doing okay, but make no mistake, I thought about not getting out of bed a lot of mornings. I cried all the way to work on many days and cried all the way home. I had constant flashbacks of the moment Jesse died. Constant thoughts of not being able to say goodbye. Instead, be happy that you helped your friend or family through the worst day of their lives and hope that you don't have to be repaid any time soon. I was grateful to my friends; I was just not always capable of expressing my thanks.

"You're taking this better than I expected." To be honest, I personally didn't mind hearing this statement. I knew people were curious about what they perceived as my strength. You have to remember that, in many cases, they were seeing me for the first time three months after my son died. While they were on Day 1, I was on Day 90. I had had some time to think about things other than my son's death. I wasn't always that strong. I was surviving.

For example, for three months after Jesse died, my profile picture on social media was a picture of him. I agonized over changing it back to a photo of myself, but I was worried about what people would think. Would they think I was crass? That I had moved on? That I was a bad parent? I didn't want to be judged because I was riddled with guilt. Sometimes this phrase will be taken well; other times it may not, depending on where a person's mind is at.

"God doesn't give you more than you can handle." I thought a lot about this one. At the time of Jesse's death, I didn't care what God wanted. I wasn't even sure a God existed. All I knew was that I was in pain. As time healed me, I realized that people always meant well when they said this.

***

A year after Jesse died, I received a caring note from one of the nurses that worked on him. When I got the note, I cried as I recalled a different nurse who had forgotten why she had come into Jesse's room. My memory of that nurse was not a positive one. In fact, my clearest memory of her was that when she entered the hospital room that was filled with people saying goodbye to a beautiful 13-year-old boy, another nurse asked her how her day had been going. In front of all of us she said, "It's been pretty good so far."

For a year, I had thought many times about reaching out to her and telling her how those words had affected me. Turns out, I didn't have to. She reached out to me. She actually sent me a note. I don't have the note any longer, but I did send her a response:

> Hi Cheryl,
> Thank you for your note in the mail today about Jesse. It has been a very long year for us and we do our best to remember him in ways he would be proud. I've written a book about grief since Jesse died that is on its way to a publisher. It's about surviving the first six months, how to deal with people's reactions and questions and how to help those around us know what is appropriate and inappropriate.
>
> On March 25 of last year, another family lost their 14-year-old to type 1 diabetes. I didn't know them then, but they have since become very important people in my life. We even journeyed together for 105 miles on our bikes in Death Valley this past October in honor of our sons. She works as an ER nurse and, since losing her son, has struggled to work efficiently without thinking of what happened to her own child while she sees death all around her day in and day out. We've

had long discussions about how difficult it must be to work as a nurse and witness the deaths of children, and how she needs to shut off emotionally in order to go home to her own family at night and behave normally.

On the other hand, I think it's important that I express my feelings about what happened the day my son died. This has been eating away at me for a long time. That day is still a blur. The pain and anguish were beyond anyone's comprehension. Compassion was so important. The lead detective from that day has become a close friend to me after she got to know who Jesse was. The firefighters and other first responders have become friends too. I reached out to everyone who was affected by the events of that day because I know now what it feels like to lose someone. I know that it must be difficult for nurses too.

With that said, I honestly don't remember all the nurses that helped that day. I have always wanted to reach out but was unsure which nurse was the one whose behavior has bothered me to this day. To the nurse who was pushing fluids through my dying son's arm as his entire family and friends sobbed around him trying to let him go....leaning

> over to the new nurse on the shift and telling her you were having a pretty good day so far was a callous and thoughtless comment. Your pretty good day was the worst day of my life — a day that I have had to relive in my mind over and over while I watch healthy 14-year-old boys live day after day. Your pretty good day should have been discussed outside our room. And while my soul is full of forgiveness, and I've accepted what was given to me in this life, I must say that the nursing staff should be reminded frequently to remember where they are standing, that lives are changed forever in those rooms and a thoughtless statement like that can remain in a person's mind forever.
>
> I do not remember the name of the nurse who said it, but, for all I know, Cheryl, it could have been you. I'm not writing this out of hate or blame. I say it so the next family who comes through there is treated respectfully and with kindness.

To be honest, I don't remember her reaction to the note. I don't even remember if she reached out to respond to my comments, but I didn't care. Jesse's life mattered, and I wanted her to remember not to say those words in front of the next family.

MICHELLE BAUER

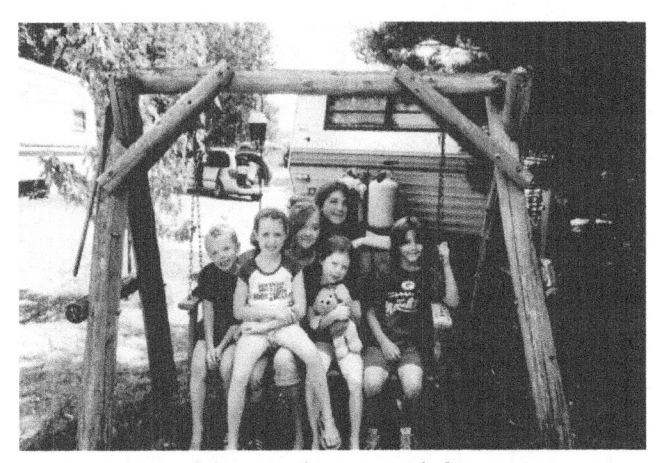

Jesse and the annual picture with his cousins

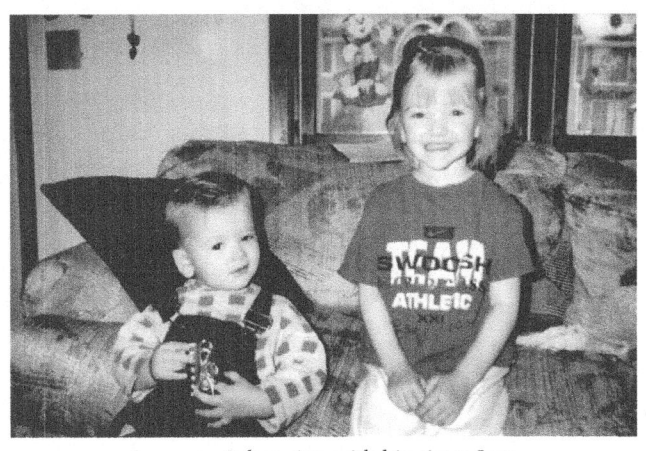

Jesse, age 2, hanging with big sister Sam

15
How Many Kids do you Have?
(Written over several months following Jesse's death)

> *"You never know how strong you are until being strong is the only choice you have."*
> *-Bob Marley*

I KNEW THE DAY WOULD COME. I KNEW I'D HAVE to get back out there eventually and re-enter the world. I figured I'd run into lots of well-meaning people. However, I wasn't always prepared for people who were disrespectful or just plain ignorant. These are some of the questions I was asked over and over again.

"How many kids do you have?" For the first month or so, when people asked this question, it felt like they were sticking a knife in me. I was so sad all the time and hesitant to even go out in public for fear of hearing questions like this. As time passed, it became less and less painful. Why? I think it was because of sheer repetition. I talked about Jesse so much that sometimes it was if somebody else was actually doing the speaking.

I found that the best way for me to answer this question was by saying, "It depends." For instance, if it was a random person that I didn't plan on getting to know, my answer was, "Three." I left it at that. An example that happened more than once was when I would check out at the grocery store with lots of kid-related items, the clerk might say, "Wow, how many kids do you have?" I realized she was just trying to be nice and there was no reason for me to have to go through the pain of explaining again. Nor was it fair to dump on a total stranger.

There were plenty of other times when I was in random conversations and the question would be asked, "So, how many kids do you have?" I would usually answer, "Three." If the person was invested in getting to know me and asked about their ages, I would decide if it was worth my time to go into details. My answer would typically be, "Nine, thirteen and sixteen." Of course, I realized I couldn't always say this knowing that Jesse would forever be thirteen. I knew someday I would figure out the best answer.

If more questions followed, and if it felt right, I'd say, "Joey is nine, Samantha is sixteen, but my son Jesse died a few months ago at thirteen." I realized that when I said this, I was almost forcing the person to make an investment in me. Hello, 800 lb. gorilla in the room! I tried to be nice and polite and found myself actually comforting some people. I also found that some people were honestly interested, so if I was strong myself, I actually helped them get through the conversation. I spoke of pride and love and about how much we missed Jesse. It was never my intent to drown others in my sorrow, but I'll be honest, there were times when I let it all out, maybe just to punish the person for asking. Kind of like, "You asked! Well, here you go, partner, have at it." I'm not perfect.

You'll have to develop your own flowchart of answers and get ready for the general public.

"You are so strong; I don't know how you do it." No one ever meant ill toward me when they said this. They were admiring me for my strength and my courage. After all, I was the one who had experienced this loss, not them. They didn't know that I was in pain a lot of times, especially at first when I was literally living moment to moment. How could they possibly know what it had been like? And why would I want them to understand and feel what I felt?

I always answered this question by saying, "You don't know what strong is until strong is your only option." It's true, isn't it? What were my options? Curl up in a ball on my bed? Couldn't. I had to live my life. My heart was left with a gaping hole, but there were others in my life who needed me. Sometimes I would say, "I'm not strong. I'm just living how I have to, to get through my days."

"So what's new?" I heard this innocent question many times. I recall going to the Juvenile Diabetes Research Foundation gala, an event in town where most people knew me and knew what happened to Jesse. That night I ran into someone I hadn't seen since a bike ride in California in 2005. He was a friend of some people who probably should have told him what had happened, yet he was unaware. He approached me and we started a conversation. So many things went through my mind but mainly this thought: "My God, he has no clue what happened, and I have to tell him." As soon as I said, "You know Jesse died, right?" his face went white and he genuinely didn't know what to say. The pain of that moment was harder on me because, while I was about 70 days into my grieving process, this conversation was bringing me right back to Day 1, whether I liked it or not.

Jesse's dad found himself having a similar conversation a few months into the grieving process. On the cul-de-sac where we raised our kids together, we had a strong bond with most of the neighbors. Over the years in our quiet little neighborhood, we would wheel a firepit into the middle of the street – a sure indicator that the neighbors were ready to bring out some chairs and sit by the fire while the kids played games or one of the dads put on a scary mask and chased them as they half-laughed, half-screamed. The nights were filled with so much laughter.

On this night, shortly after Jesse's death, a neighbor from up the street walked down. He wasn't the kind of guy that came out frequently, but when he did he always inquired about the kids and always had something cool to give Jesse. On this occasion he came down the street to the firepit and quickly said, "Hey, I haven't seen Jesse around lately, but I thought he might like this. Gotta run." Jesse's dad stood with his mouth open thinking many thoughts. He knew he should stop him and tell him. The neighbors stood there quietly, probably kicking themselves for not taking the time to tell him that Jesse was gone.

Months went by and the Fourth of July was upon us. Despite the fact that I had gotten divorced and moved, the neighbors invited us back for the celebration. I was happy to see everyone. That same neighbor who had previously talked to Jesse's dad and was still unaware of his death pulled up on his motorcycle as I was casually speaking with someone. With a smile, he went on and on about how excited his nephew was to hang out with Jesse for the fireworks. He also said he had some things for Jesse but hadn't seen him around. I gulped. Literally. I saw the other neighbors looking on in horror, wondering how I would answer him. There was no knight in shining armor ready to save this damsel. I was going to have to tell him. Yes, it was awkward, but I said, "Steve, I'm so sorry, but Jesse died in February." He looked terribly sad and said, "What happened?" I could see tears on his face. I told him the news in my "I've already said this a million times" voice, but it still hurt like hell to tell this man who really didn't know. He was devastated, and I walked away feeling sad and hurt again, pushed back in time to the day Jesse died. I didn't want to hurt like that anymore.

"How did he die?" I rarely ran into people who were just trying to snoop by asking this question. In fact, sometimes it seemed like this question would pop out of a person's mouth before he or she was ready to hear the answer.

> *These are some of the questions*
> *I was asked over and over again.*

At first I found it excruciating to tell people what happened mainly because I didn't want to relive those horrible moments. I just wasn't ready. Over time, I was able to get through it more easily. Most people asked general questions, and due to the nature of his death and the fact that I was so active in the diabetes community, it was a natural question for parents who feared the same consequences for their own children. For them, I completely understood.

If I cared about the people asking, I told them everything they wanted to know. I found it strangely cathartic to explain what had happened over and over again, especially when I knew the people cared about me and really were concerned about what had happened to Jesse.

At the same time, there were those who pushed it too far with me, at least in my mind. They wanted all the gory details.

For instance, after Jesse's death I went on a national news show to talk about what had happened. I made a point in this case to know my audience. I knew that moms and dads of kids with diabetes weren't ready to hear that a child could actually die from this disease. So I made a point to say it was a tragedy, that even Jesse would tell them and their children to continue living their lives to the fullest. Yet, I was bombarded with questions from a couple of women who seemed to want the answer to be that I was a bad parent, that I must have done something wrong, that I was the cause of my own son's death. I realized, however, that the reason they were projecting blame on me was to make themselves feel less afraid for their own kids' mortality.

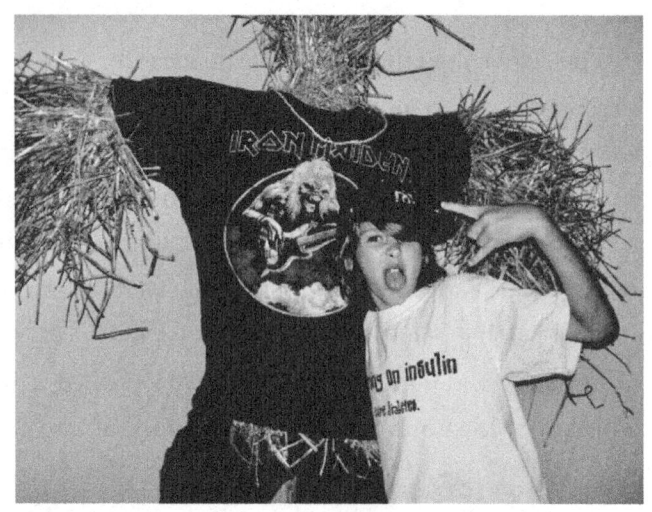

Jesse, age 13, fooling around at the water park

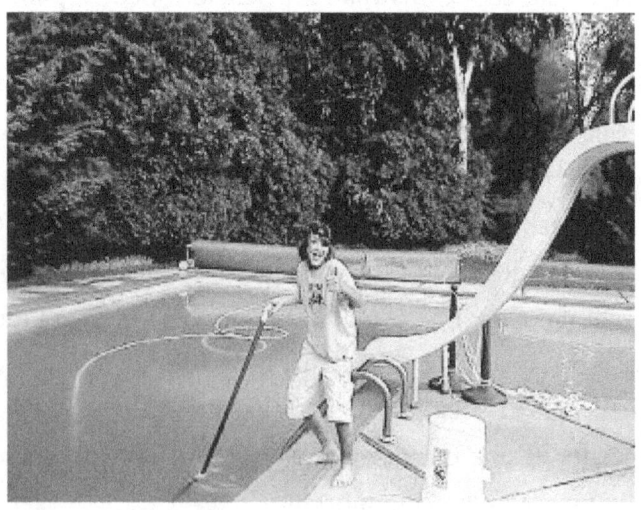

Jesse, age 13, cleaning the backyard pool

16
A Guide for Family and Friends

(Written over time after Jesse's death)

> *"Every single time you help someone stand up, you are helping humanity rise."*
> -Steve Maraboli

ON THE DAY JESSE DIED, I CLEARLY REMEMber calling a handful of people. I called my friend Sandy. I wanted her to be there to help me. The next person I called was Amy, somebody who had been a lifelong friend and part of my support system. Lastly, I called a co-worker to make sure my friends at work were updated. Why did I do that? I think I had gone into some sort of "protect myself" mode knowing that I was going to need some help. Julia, my neighbor who was always there for me, called me next, out of the blue.

I can't imagine what was going through all of their heads. They didn't know what to do either, but somehow they figured it out. They picked me up and didn't let me fall. I learned a lot of great lessons from my wonderful friends that day during the following weeks, months and years. There are a lot of things people can do to help others who are suffering through a tragedy like losing a child.

Be present. Don't look for excuses not to help. I knew it was hard; I knew it was difficult for my friends to deal with what happened to me, but I needed them like never before. Even when I said, "I don't want anyone around," I really did. It was necessary. Other people will need the same type of support that I was given. Be ready to give it.

> *There were times when I didn't even know what I needed help with. I was just grateful when people jumped in and started helping.*

Set up a memorial fund. Especially with the loss of a child, chances are that many families do not have money put aside to pay for a funeral and the other expenses that go along with it. Don't ask; just DO. Get a memorial fund started so people have a place to donate immediately.

Plan a memorial event. It may have seemed sudden, but

for us it was not only cathartic to be with so many people who loved Jesse after his funeral, but it also helped raise a lot of funds.

Help with funeral planning. We needed help finding and securing a funeral home; we needed help with funds to pay for the funeral and we also needed help finding a church in which to have the funeral.

Let them talk and talk and talk and talk. The more we talked and grieve, the better we felt.

Answer the grieving person's phone for them. Taking calls and talking on the phone was exhausting. Of course people meant well, but having to tell the story over and over was brutal and painful.

Plan the food at the funeral luncheon. We had so many people that made and served food after the funeral. It was a small but extremely lovely gesture on the part of our friends and family.

Put a slide show together or make some picture boards. It was difficult to go through old photos of Jesse. It meant a lot to have help with this activity.

Put away items of the person they love. When Jesse died, there were so many little reminders of his presence all over our house. It was helpful to me when somebody collected many of those things and tucked them away so I could go through them later. There was no need to box up his belongings. That could be saved for another day.

Call and offer help, or just start helping. There were times when I didn't even know what I needed help with. I was just grateful when people jumped in and started helping.

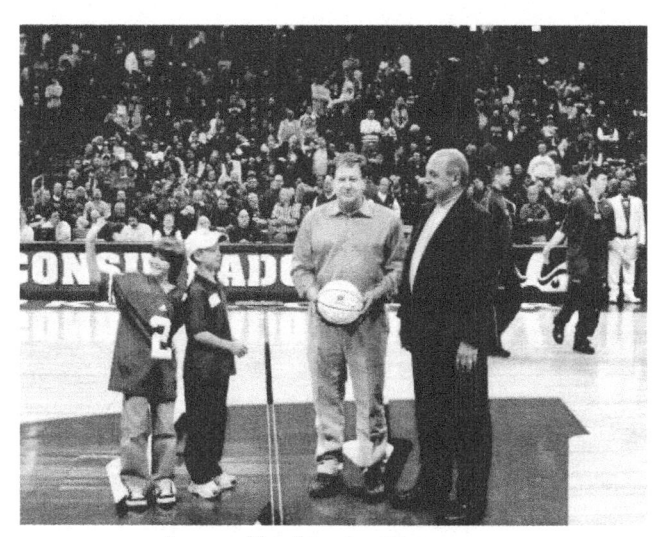

Jesse and his friend getting a game
ball from Coach Alvarez

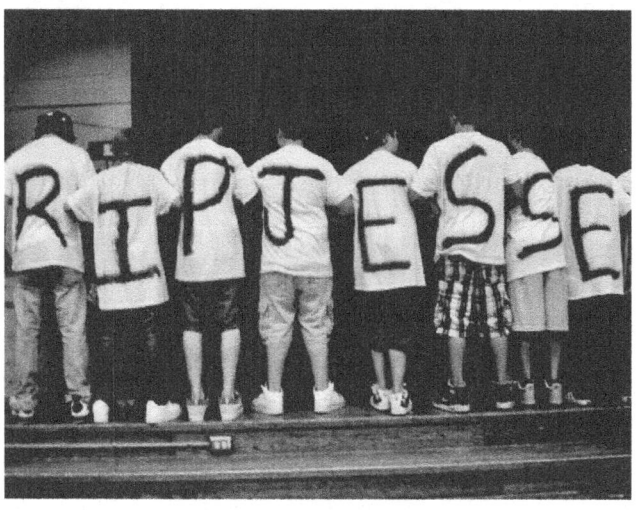

Jesse's classmates at Toki Middle
School showing their love

How Jesse Was Here Came to Be

DURING THE SUMMER OF 2009, I DECIDED to take my kids on a little family vacation to a nearby campground for a long weekend. We spent the weekend swimming, jumping on trampolines, paddle boating and roasting marshmallows. In the evenings, we would go over to the bar on the property, and I use the term 'bar' loosely. It was really nothing more than an oversized shed with a portable bar, bar tables and stools. The kids loved going there because they were handed gold metallic markers with only one rule - don't write on the ceiling. The kids giggled as they wrote all over the walls.

Days after Jesse's death, for no reason that I can remember, it popped into my head that every summer the campground probably had to paint over all of that artwork. For some reason, that thought made me very emotional. It was almost as if by painting over the words my son wrote – **Jesse Was Here** – they were erasing him from his time on earth.

Members of my family went to work. We contacted the campground and established an agreement that we would pay them to let us remove what Jesse had written and then repair the hole in the wall. We got some bad news shortly thereafter. My family let me know that it would be impossible to remove Jesse's writing because the property was in foreclosure, locked up and owned by the bank.

At the time, I just accepted it as fate, thinking there was nothing I could do about it. Then, a small miracle. A couple of weeks later, a 12" x 12" cutout of the words Jesse wrote on the wall of that bar was sitting on my dining room table. And that's all I can say about that.

That piece of wall with Jesse's words written on it sat in my dining room for several years as a quiet reminder that he once sat in that room. As the years passed, a friend of mine asked about it one day and said, "It deserves more. Would you mind if I made a case for it?" He built a beautiful frame for it that housed not only the piece of the wall but a picture we had found of Jesse actually writing the words.

As time moved forward, I could never bring myself to hang it on the wall of that house. The honest truth was that I didn't feel it was home. I was still a single mom, renting a house, and it felt too permanent to hang it on a wall at that time.

In 2017, when Jeff and I started to look at buying a home together, we fell in love with one particular house. Upon entering the front door, we could hardly believe our eyes.

Right in the entryway was a space, perfectly carved out, with the exact measurements we needed to hang Jesse's frame. It was the perfect spot for it.

We bought that house and moved in. When you enter our home, it's the first thing you see. Once I settled into this house with Jeff, I finally felt like I was home.

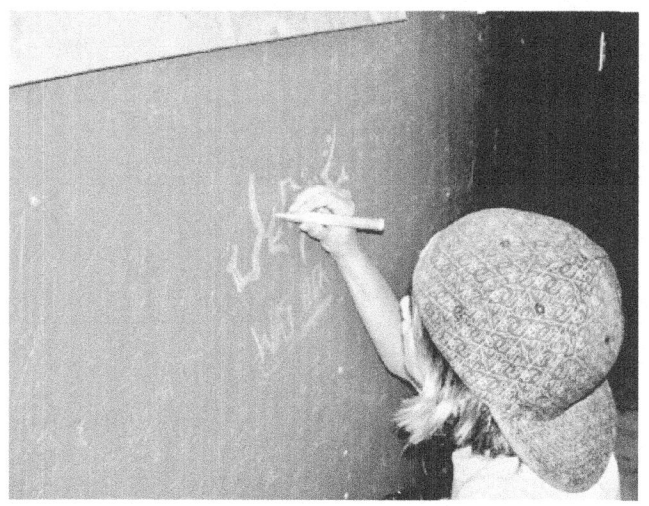

Jesse, age 12, writing his famous words

Epilogue

"At times, our own light goes out and is rekindled by a spark from another person. Each of us has cause to think with deep gratitude of those who have lighted the flame within us."
-Albert Einstein

IT'S BEEN QUITE A JOURNEY TO GET TO THE END of this story. What I've learned, however, is there really is no end to our story.

There were times while I was writing various parts of this book when I worried I would forget his face, forget his voice, forget my memories of him. A decade later, I promise you, I still see that smirk on his face, I still hear his squeaky giggle. I can still see in my mind the day I told him not to post on social media about the moment when we all realized that Dorothy, his hamster, had male parts. I yelled from the dining room into the living room, "Jesse Thomas, take that off social media!" The shout was answered with giggles, "okay,

okay, mom." I sat chuckling as I read his corrected version: "I had a great day at school today. My hamster has balls. Is that better, Mom?"

As I re-read those words and reflect on that day, memories like that still make me smile, but they also bring back the pain of knowing that those were the last words he ever put out into the world. No, those memories will never leave me.

I had a lot of shit in my life with Jesse in it, and I have a lot of good in my life with Jesse gone. Seems unfair, doesn't it? While 2010 was the worst year of my life, I flash forward to my life in 2020 – a life that is filled with amazing old friends who stood by me through the worst of times. Then there are the new people I've met along the journey and collected as friends who always say, "I really wish I could have met Jesse."

No one says that more than my husband, Jeff. I'm fortunate to have met him when I was ready to open up and allow joy back into my life.

From the beginning, he tried to get into my head and understand what made me tick. I was unaware of it at the time, but he would take notes about my friends, my siblings and my favorite foods along with important information to remember about my kids. I still can't imagine dating somebody (like me) who had traveled to the deepest, darkest place in her soul and then climbed out. Yet, this man, who only knows my son through my stories, my pictures and sometimes my inconsolable crying at night, chose to love me anyway.

It felt appropriate to end this version of my story with something I said earlier in this book, about how I would never take another family photo because my family was forever broken. That also meant no blathering, happy holiday cards detailing all the joys of life.

And then it happened. A year ago, when Jeff and I made the decision to get married, we knew the most important thing was to join our two families together and have only them present. After climbing to the top of the state capitol in Madison and leaving behind a small memory of Jesse at the spot where we married, we descended to the front steps together to start the next chapter of the story. And we took a family picture.

In the end, no family picture is ever going to be perfect. It can't be because it's always in the moment. Our lives will always have loss, some expected, chronological. Other losses will be untimely and shocking, literally taking our breath away.

We can only continue to embrace those around us while we are together and eventually remember that they, too, were here.

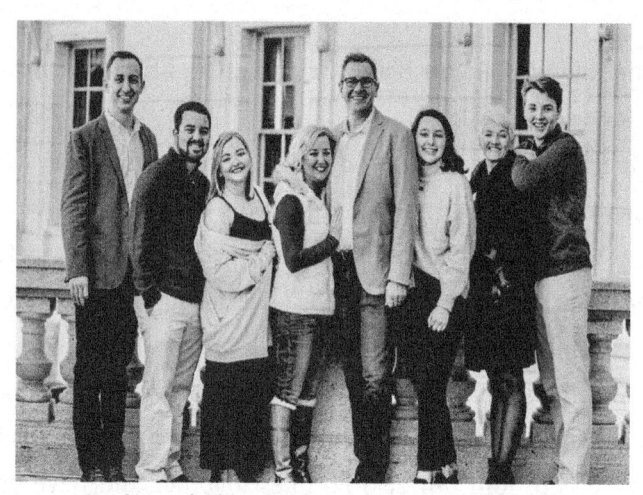

Our beautiful blended family on our wedding day,
December 17, 2018, on the steps of the Capitol

Resources

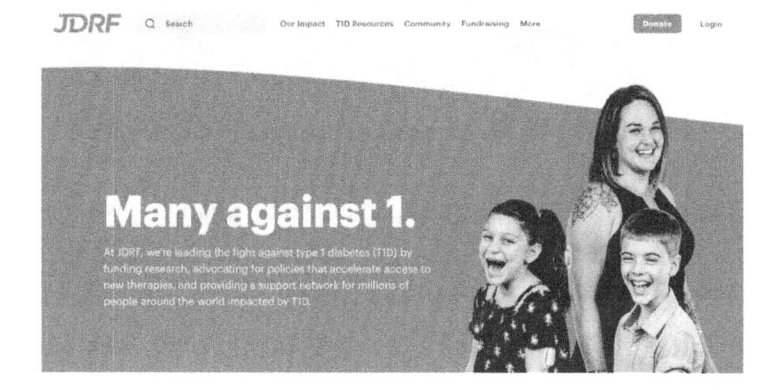

JDRF is leading the fight against type 1 diabetes (T1D) by funding research, advocating for policies that accelerate access to new therapies and providing a support network for millions of people around the world impacted by T1D.

www.jdrf.org

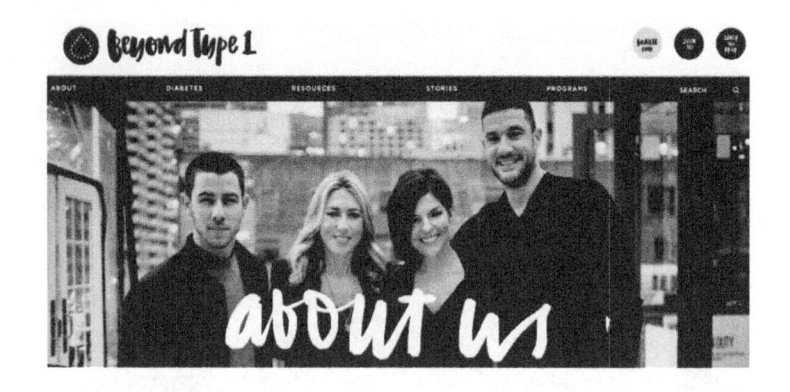

Beyond Type 1 is a nonprofit organization changing what it means to live with diabetes. Through platforms, programs, resources and grants, Beyond Type 1 is uniting the global diabetes community and providing solutions to improve lives today.

www.beyondtype1.org

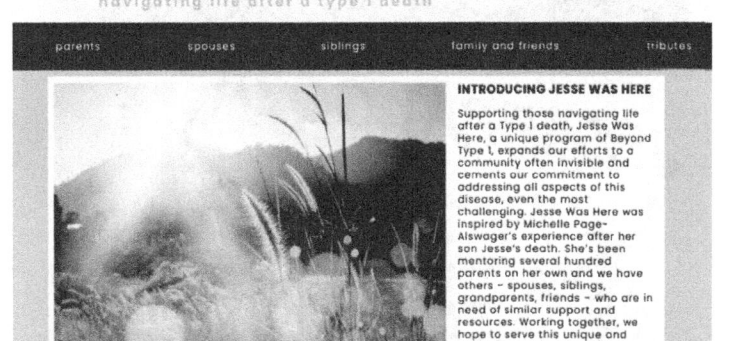

Jesse Was Here is a program run by Beyond Type 1 and supported by JDRF. Inspired by Michelle Bauer after she lost her son to type 1 diabetes, Jesse Was Here serves as a mentoring program for spouses, siblings, grandparents and friends in the diabetes community who have lost loved ones.

www.jesse-was-here.org

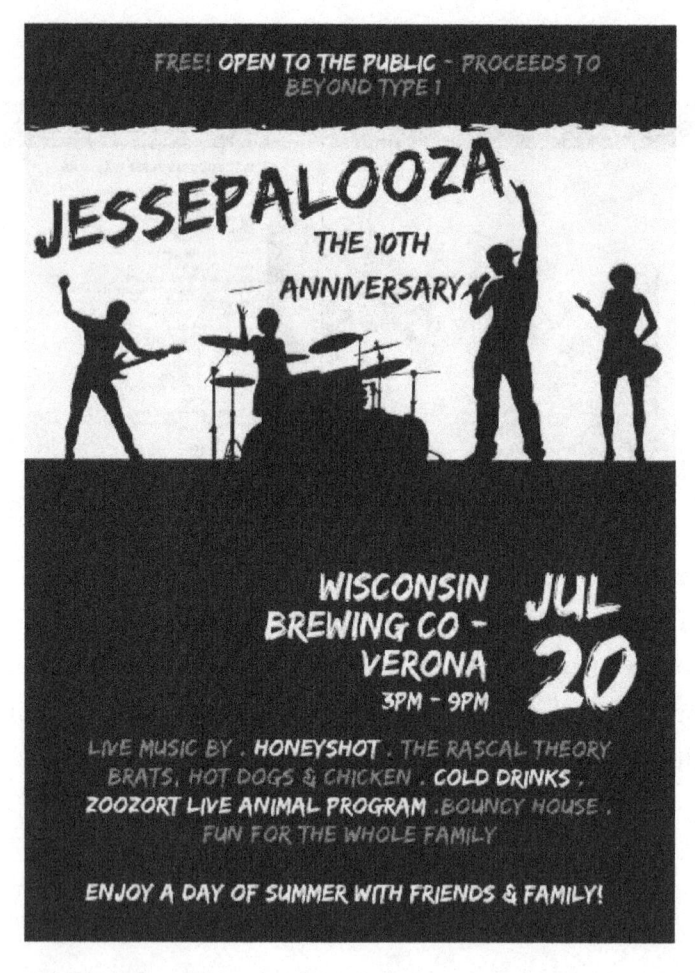

JESSEPALOOZA is the annual music festival held in honor of Jesse in Madison, Wisconsin. Proceeds benefit the program Jesse Was Here at Beyond Type 1.

JDRF Ride to Cure Diabetes

THE JDRF RIDE TO CURE DIABETES IS SOMEthing I've done every year since 2004 for my son. Jesse was very proud of my first ride in Death Valley, the first time I had ever ridden 100 miles on my bike.

Since losing Jesse to type 1 diabetes on 2/3/2010, at the age of 13, JDRF has embraced not only the loss of Jesse but the loss of many others. To commemorate these loved ones, we have incorporated a mile of silence at mile 23 (2/3) of each ride.

We ride 99 miles to celebrate the accomplishments and milestones we've reached in finding a cure; we ride 1 mile in silence to remember all those we've lost. Help me remember my 1.

Did You Know?

Did you know that T1D
- is an autoimmune disease in which a person's pancreas stops producing insulin, the hormone that controls blood sugar levels?
- strikes children and adults suddenly and is unrelated to diet and lifestyle?
- requires constant daily carb counting, blood-glucose testing and lifelong dependence on insulin?
- is a constant balancing act that can result in stress and sleepless nights?

There is no way to prevent T1D and there is no cure – yet. JDRF is working hard to change that. JDRF has played a key role in the discovery and availability of nearly every major T1D advance over the past 50 years. For the first time in our history, there is a clear path to cures for T1D. Decades of research have brought us to a transformative moment where scientific advances are being turned into therapies that are changing the course of T1D. Together we must drive as many of these therapies to market as quickly as we can.

Every dollar you donate helps fund research for breakthroughs to help everyone with T1D live healthier and longer lives, until this disease no longer exists.

We can't get to the finish line without you.

MICHELLE BAUER

IF YOU WOULD LIKE TO DONATE:

www.ride.jdrf.org

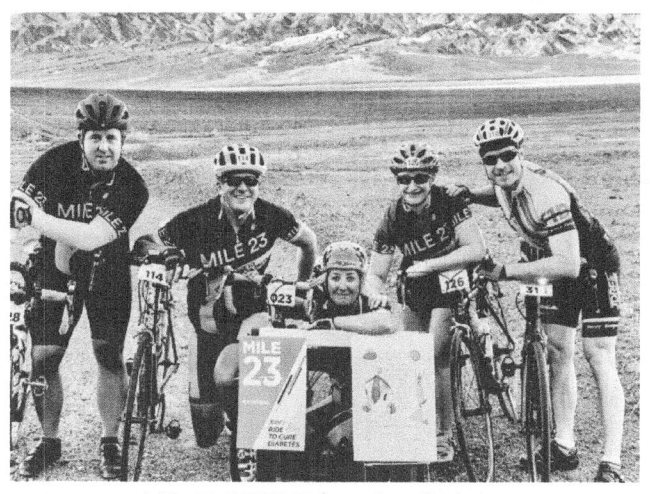

Mile 23, JDRF Ride to Cure Diabetes

Memories

I RECEIVED THIS NOTE JUST THREE WEEKS AFTER Jesse's funeral. I was sitting at my dining room table, sobbing, not knowing what I was going to do with my life, when this arrived with a note from his teacher. She said, "Jesse could write about anything in this essay." He chose to talk about all the things I had done for him in the world of diabetes – this, the boy, who always said, "Mom! Stop talking about diabetes!"

JESSE WAS HERE

Student ID # 7 3 7 0 2

DAY 3: Write Final Copy

Writing Prompts

CHECK (✓) the box next to the prompt you have chosen.

☑ **Explanatory:** Identify someone who has courage. This person may be someone you know or someone who is famous. Explain what makes this person courageous by describing what he or she does to inspire you.

☐ **Persuasive:** Some research suggests that using electronic devices such as video games, cell phones, and iPods interferes with learning. Do you agree or disagree? Use your experiences and observations to persuade your audience of your position.

☐ **Open:** Write an essay that explains, persuades and/or describes a subject of your choice from your personal knowledge or experience.

- Today you will have 45 minutes to write your final copy. Please write as neatly as possible.
- Revise and edit your writing in the green Draft Booklet. You may use the dictionary and thesaurus. Use the Writer's Checklist on the cover to help you.
- Write your final copy on the pages in this White Final Copy Booklet. Add extra paper if you need it.
- Proofread and make corrections before submitting. If you make a mistake, you may cross out or add words to your final copy without starting over.

Begin your final copy here.

My mom is a very courageous person. She does many things to show how courageous she is. She always does brave things to make my life easier, even if they are difficult.

My mom's name is Michelle Alswager. She always does things to help me. One of the biggest things is she applied for a job at J.D.R.F, a place where they raise money for research about diabetes. She got the job and helped a lot in the community.

My Mom is also courageous for her athletisism. In 2006, she began intense training to bike one-hundred and five miles in Death Valley, California.

She would bike sixty-five miles every week about three times. She went to Death Valley and completed the one-hundred and five miles in the desert. She enjoyed it so much that she did it four more times!

Then she wanted a harder challenge. She decided to attempt Ironman Madison, WI, a triathalon. Except she couldn't swim, and she didn't run. But that did not stop her. She began swimming lessons and started running. She finnished Ironman on time. I was so proud!

She is currently is working on making a documentary. It is about people with diabetes doing Ironman. She is working so hard on it. It is almost done. The documentary has taken about two years of filming, and will play around the world in Film Festivals when it is done.

This year my mom got a new job at Brava Magazine. She wanted this job so much! Unfortunately Brava closed down because the owner didn't want it. But my mom gathered her co-workers and planned a way to save the business. They found a new owner and saved Brava. These are some reasons why my mom is a very courageous person!

JESSE WAS HERE

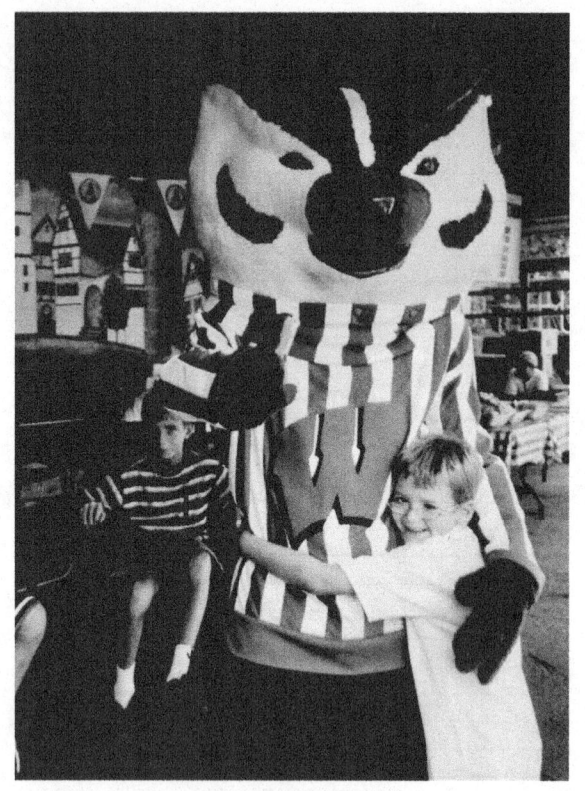

Jesse, age 7, with Bucky Badger at Backyard Bash,
an event we created to raise money for JDRF

MICHELLE BAUER

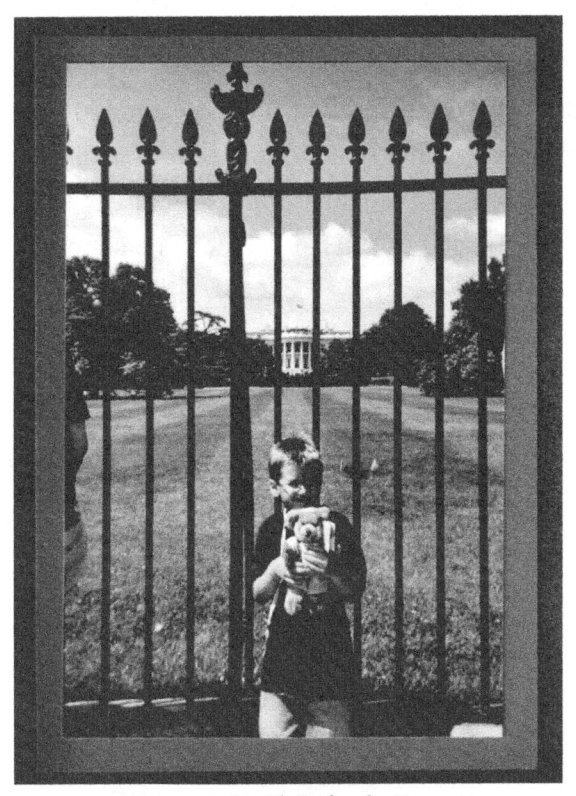

Jesse, age 6, with Rufus the Bear,
who also has type 1 diabetes

These last four pictures were taken at the same time, when Jesse was six years old. In 2003, Jesse took part in the JDRF Children's Congress which brought together 200 kids with type 1 diabetes from all over the world to speak to their representatives on Capitol Hill. Jesse and two other delegates met with all of the legislators including Senator Herb Kohl and Representative Tammy Baldwin. They appeared before a Senate hearing advocating for more funds for diabetes research. Our family took advantage of that time to do a fundraiser. We sold cookbooks with a picture of Jesse on the cover and donated $20,000 to our local chapter of JDRF.

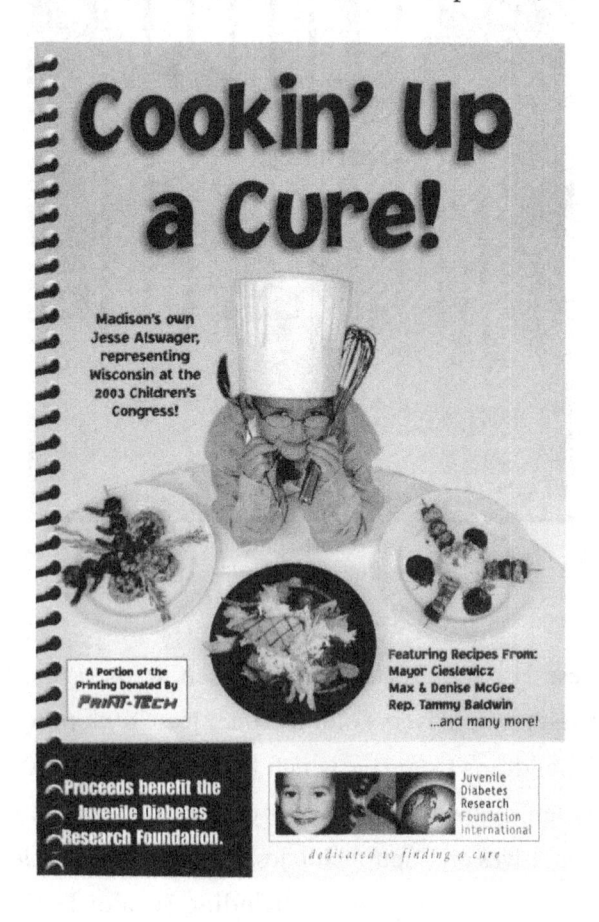

MICHELLE BAUER

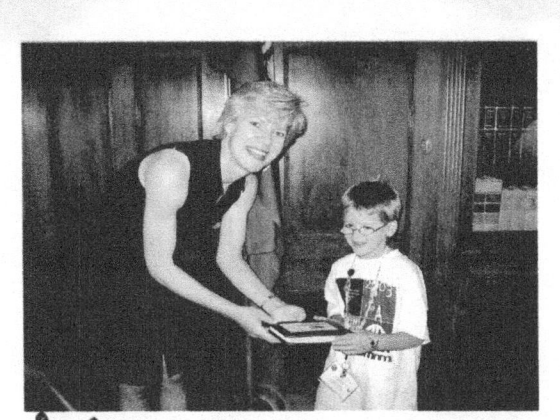

Dear Jesse,
Thanks for being such a great advocate!
Tammy Baldwin

Jesse, age 6, with then Representative Tammy Baldwin

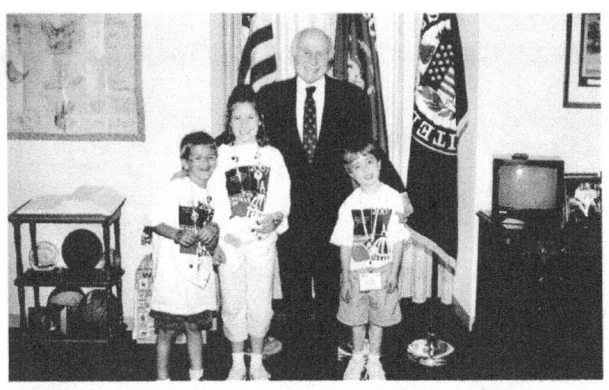

To my friend, Jesse Alswager, from
Herb Kohl

Jesse, age 6, with then Senator Herb Kohl

Life Sentence
by Joe Brady

Did I say these words to a hundred,
a thousand parents?

"My name is Michelle Alswager
and my son, like your child, has type 1 diabetes
but don't worry, it's not a death sentence."

My son Jesse, so little, diagnosed at age three
and so early gone at thirteen.
I ask myself, what will I tell the parents now?
With eyes closed, I see my son…and know the answer:

Refuse with me to feel sorry for him
For he lived his diagnosis as a life sentence
with no time limit guarantee.

A life sentence to celebrate his days
touching others with his smile and patient ways,
chilling with his school friends and neighbors,

advocating with Governor, Congress,
and doctors to find the cure.

Hanging with Dad at neighborhood parties
loving music, playing his sweet-sounding life melody
carving sharp, crisp lines with Sean on snowy slopes
laughing with brother and sisters at mom's corny jokes.

For him, beating the disease was to never
compromise, yield, submit or succumb
to an affliction whose victories
are counted with each lost possibility and
"Can't do 'cause I've got type 1."

Never did he say, "pity me" or "it's not fair."
Instead we heard "what's next?" and "let's go" and "cool!"
as he lived his life sentence.

So please hear me, dear parent with
newly diagnosed type 1,
not once did my son yield, submit or succumb.
His life was rich, vibrant, a celebration…
Jesse didn't lose – he won.

Joe Brady is the cycling coach and leader of the JDRF Ride to Cure Diabetes, Western Wisconsin Chapter

About the Author

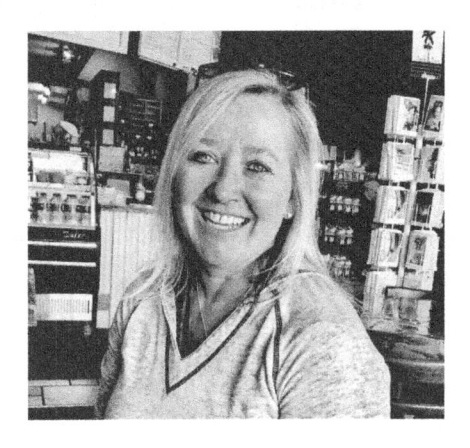

MICHELLE HAS BEEN A STRONG ADVOcate in the "d" world since her son Jesse was diagnosed with Type 1 diabetes in 2000 at the age of three. After the sudden loss of her son at the age of 13, she continued to advocate, educate and push the envelope in her son's name. Michelle is the founder and executive producer of the documentary *The Science of Inspiration: Diabetes and Athletes* – otherwise known as *Triabetes* – about 12 athletes with diabetes completing an Ironman triathlon. Her diabetes credits include working as a moderator on the JDRF

Online Diabetes Support Team and as an executive director for two diabetes organizations. She also participates each year in the JDRF Ride to Cure Diabetes. She is currently the Sales Director for Thrivable, where she helps diabetes related companies conduct research, and a member of Beyond Type 1's own Leadership Council. In addition to spending a lot of time on her road bike, Michelle is a three-time IRONMAN finisher. In fact, she raced with the ROI Endurance Team at IRONMAN Wisconsin in 2015. In her spare time she also works with Beyond Type 1's program called *Jesse Was Here*. The program offers support to families across the world who have lost loved ones to Type 1 diabetes. Michelle lives in Madison, Wisconsin, with her husband, Jeff, and their combined six children. This is Michelle's first book.

Made in the USA
Monee, IL
15 November 2024